THE FITNESS BIBLE

THE FITNESS BIBLE

by

LAW PAYNE, PATRICIA PAYNE,
DUSTIN BOSWELL, LESLIE BOSWELL

THE FITNESS BIBLE

by
Law Payne, Patricia Payne,
Dustin Boswell, Leslie Boswell

TABLE OF CONTENTS

Dear Heavenly Father,

Every day, we have important life changing decisions and actions to make and we humbly ask that you give us the patience to await your answers and guidance. We have prayed consistently and diligently allowing faith to take over. Allow our minds to be still as you work out every situation for us Lord, for you make all things work together for our good and your time is the perfect time. For, with your guidance, anything is possible.

Amen

DEFINING HEALTH AND A BALANCED WEIGHT

The term health implies a disease-free state. It is also connected to a state of wellness, that is, how you think and perceive about other things. Being healthy means being positive and making rigorous efforts and smart choices.

Weight and health are connected in innumerable ways. An overweight person is susceptible to so many diseases like diabetes, heart stroke, high blood pressure, breathing problems, gout including others. Thus, before taking on a new diet schedule, it is always recommended to consult a doctor.

WHEN ARE YOU OVERWEIGHT?

There are many ways to know the point when your weight departs from the optimal weight.

BMI:

Based on your weight and height, Body Mass Index helps you to know a healthy range of your weight according to your height. You can calculate it using online BMI calculators.

SKIN - FOLD THICKNESS:

Via this, you can measure the thickness of fats in your skin. It's done using 'caliper'.

WAIST TO HIP RATIO (WHR):

Accustomed with the terms of beer belly and pot belly, right? Often mocked at, these are as dangerous as any other fatty area of your body. The ratio is obtained by dividing the narrowest waist level to the widest hip level.

These 3 can be used in combos to assess if you are unhealthy. But the rule of thumb still remains as how you feel about your body.

While there is a negative relation between being overweight and being healthy, there is strong positive relation between exercising and being healthy. Exercise becomes even more important as you age. It helps in improving your metabolism. Playing sports can increase oxygen supply to your heart and you breathe better. It also helps in faster clotting process, increased heart muscles, more stable blood pressure and lowers the risk of diabetes.

MIND TOO MATTERS:

What you think and how you think also has drastic effects on your weight. Let's see how.

Depression and anxiety also need to be discussed on analyzing how mind affects your weight. There is no proper

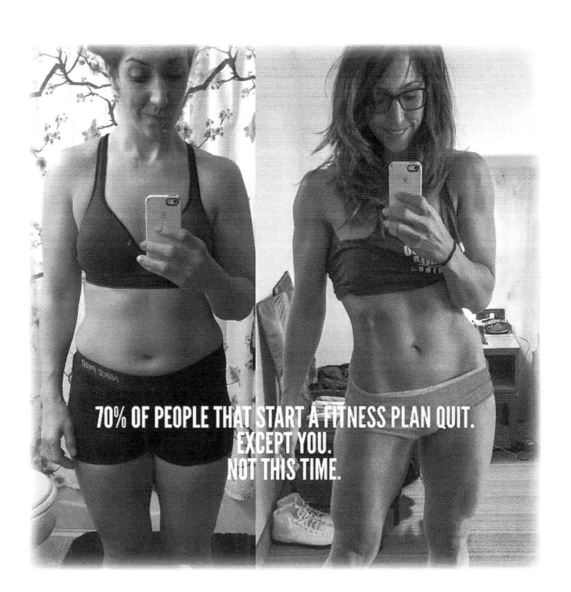

70% OF PEOPLE THAT START A FITNESS PLAN QUIT.
EXCEPT YOU.
NOT THIS TIME.

definition of depression, but it is a blah state where you lose the excitement to do anything. Depression may increase your appetite and thus make you gain weight, or it may decrease your appetite and will cause sleeping problems.

Anxiety again can make you eat more and cause sleeping disorders. It may increase your alcohol intake thus adding to your calories. Stress again fashions in the same way, with a difference that it does not come from outside; but takes birth inside you.

So all of these problems will make you turn towards eating more food or taking in liquor. Best way to get rid of these is to consult a doctor.

But the good news is a positive mind can help you in a way as no trainer or no book can. The attitude and the thought you carry can make or break you. Thus, it's wise to choose positive thought over the negative ones with a positive thinking.

Michelle is a fat person and it was difficult for her to gel with the crowd, leading to a low self-esteem. This low self-esteem madeher more negative and she ended up taking in more calories and put on more weight. Once she was made to understand how obesity was having an effect on her mind and led to more weight gain, she was more than willing to get rid of her anxieties and stress by opting for the simple tips given below.

- Replace all the 'I can'ts' with all 'I cans' and then see the miracles.
- Pen down your negative thoughts and never let them come near you again.
- Try to create positive thoughts.
- Give yourself a pat over every small achievement you have, this will increase your confidence.

WEIGHT LOSS: INTRODUCTION

Obesity is recognized as a major problem worldwide. It is the cause of many associated diseases like diabetes and some cancers. It is also one of the major reasons behind cardiac arrest, high blood pressure, stroke and breathing problems.

What most people do not know is that obesity is treatable and its effects can be reduced through a supervised weight loss. If one is obese, it is a good idea to seek professional help to reduce weight in order to have a better lifestyle and reduce one's exposure to associated diseases.

The first hurdle to overcoming obesity is recognizing the problem. Many obese people remain in denial all their lives refusing to admit that they have a problem. The second hurdle is accepting the fact that obesity can be treated. The key to overcoming obesity lies in a prudent mix of short and long term goals. This will enable you to pause at each juncture and re-evaluate your results and adjust your program to keep you in track of your ultimate goal of weight loss.

Knowing you have a problem and believing that you will lose weight is the most important factor in a weight loss program. Those people, who begin a weight loss regime with a lot of enthusiasm with the hope of quick results, may only end up crashing out of the program as quickly as they got into it.

If you are serious about weight loss, you need to have a lot of faith along with the determination to complete the program. If you are fickle-minded and have the tendency to become disheartened very quickly, you will need to have a backup plan to avoid ending the program prematurely.

In order to sustain your interest in weight loss, you need to become involved. One of the best ways to do this is by feeding your curiosity and educating yourself about every step along the way. Ask as many questions to yourself as you can in order to understand your problem better. When you ask questions, the scope of the problem diminishes. You understand which problems you do not have to worry about and recognize those you have to work on. The answers can help you focus on your immediate needs and seek help appropriately.

Search for others with similar problems. Social interactions dilute the stress associated with recognition of obesity as a problem or even in the midst of a weight loss program.

When you discuss the pros and cons of weight loss with your friends or family, and even strangers having similar problems who you may have met at a social meet or in your neighborhood, the determination to lose weight in a practical way becomes much stronger.

When you consider weight loss as an adventure to better health and lifestyle, the problem of obesity becomes more of a reason to celebrate the beginning of a new life. As always be cautious before taking the first steps and consult your doctor and have a through checkup before you begin.

GOAL SETTING AND STAYING MOTIVATED

The goals which you set should not be too easy to make you go lazy and should not be too difficult which will ultimately frustrate you. You should make S.M.A.R.T. goals which mean they should be specific, measurable, attainable, relevant and time-bound.

GETTING REAL:

It is really important to know the costs and the benefits of making such serious efforts before you finally take them on. While the costs include all the hardships and the back breaking sweat that you will put in, the benefits include a healthier life, an improved self-image, a sense of contentment and pleasure.

Thus, it is really important to know your exact motives before venturing onto a weight loss program. Because it will slowly become a part of your life! If in midway you change your goals, you will taste defeat and will feel stranded. Careful planning is all you need together with a cost benefit analysis which will help you stay motivated.

Also learn to differentiate between the long term and short term costs and benefits. While missing your routine for a day will help you laze around; but that can have drastic long term consequences. Thus, one should always weigh the costs and the benefits and then act.

SHIFTING THE SELF-IMAGE:

Losing weight is not just about losing weight, it is way of life! It will mould the way you think, your thoughts, your habits, everything. But this may take some time. Instead you should steer your mind parallel to this and try to create habits that suit your weight loss regime.

THERE CAN BE THREE SELVES:

One that we want the others to see, second is the negative self and third is the authentic or the real self. Mr. Baxter followed the stages give here and today, he has become an example of sort to all those who are trying to lose weight.

Analyze these three and come out with what your actual strengths and weaknesses are. Delve deeper into your strengths and turn your weaknesses into your strengths. Only then you will achieve what you really want. We can help you achieve your goals with our online and distant programs. Just *get in touch with us* and tread the path towards a healthier and happier life!

DIFFERENT STAGES OF CHANGE

The whole weight loss paradigm will change you slowly and steadily. It's not a one step process; but has various stages as given below.

PRE – CONTEMPLATION STAGE:

This is the stage when you realize why you want to lose weight, taking into account all the risk of being overweight. This needs to be done to remain motivated throughout the process.

CONTEMPLATION STAGE:

This includes the analyzing of the costs and benefits of losing weight and most importantly how are you going to lose weight. This stage prepares you mentally of the cyclone which is going to hit your life, the self- invited cyclone.

Thisis where you start thinking how to do it, how to lose weight and what needs to be done via SMART goals.

ACTION:

This is finally where you start acting, exercising, managing your diet, thinking positive etc.

MAINTENANCE:

This is where some results start getting reflected. But you can't stop! You have to complete the process until you get what you aimed for.

A last word of advice would be to realize that trying to be too harsh on yourself won't give you great results. Rather let the transition be smooth. If you start getting too strict about your exercise and your diet, though you might be energetic at the initial stages; your old habits might catch up with you at a later stage. Thus it is always advisable to take baby steps and achieve your goal.

THE ACTION:

This is the time you must have realized that you have made some really bad decisions in the past when you kept on eating fast food and accumulated calories. Now that you want to change it, please remember that only dieting or only exercise won't be of much help. You need a proper blend of sports, diet and mind.

TRACK YOUR WORK:

You must have penned some SMART goals and you must have thought about how much weight you need to put off. But it is really crucial to assess your work. Here's how you can do it.

A FOOD JOURNAL:

Yes, keeping an account of what you eat and what you don't will help you. You will think twice before having that pack of potato chips.

CALENDAR:

You need to mark on the calendar the days where you stuck to your plan and also the days where you were lazing around.

- Weigh yourself time and again: Weigh yourself at least once in a week to track if you have lost any pounds.

- Waist and Hip Ratio: Calculate this ratio, this also will help you analyze if you have achieved any success.

- Take pictures: In this world, pictures rule. So a slimmer you look in the picture; the more you will be motivated.

- Diets: It's not about starving yourself. Obviously it excludes fast food and other unhealthy foods. Before going into diet, let's see what exactly we mean by calories. These are the heat units generated by the energy produced by the foods consumed by the body. To put it in simple words, when you eat something, the body uses up what is necessary and stores the remaining as fat. Thus, your calorie intake should not be more than what you can use. So a healthy diet for a person who wants to lose weight is consuming lesser calories so that the body can spend the already existing calories that are stored as body fat.

A healthy diet is the one which is rich in vegetables and fruits and in which everything is consumed proportionally. There are no too big or too small chunks. Some very important nutrients which must be a part of your diet are:

1.   MACRONUTRIENTS

Carbohydrates

Usually carbohydrates are something which every person dreads off, thanks to the bad reputation they have earned all over the internet. But that is not correct. Carbs are as important as any other nutrient in our body. They can range from simple to complex. Glucose and fiber are the types of carbs which are required by the body to perform some specific functions and needs to be taken in optimum quantities.

It should constitute 40% -50% (20 to 250grams) of your daily intake, not more than that. You need carbs to have energy to exercise. You can't really ditch them altogether.

Proteins

Proteins again are a very critical element of one's diet. They are the building blocks of your body. It is made up of 20 amino acids, all of which you need in certain amounts to let your body work well. Covert your weight to kilograms to know how much protein you need. Then you need to multiply the result as:

Weight in kg x 0.8-1.8 gm/kg = protein gm.

Use 0.8 if you are healthy and use 1.8 if you are stressed or pregnant or sick.

Not more than 30% of your diet should be proteins.

Fats

Fatty acids are again a very important source of energy. They are composed of fat soluble vitamins like K, E, D and A which are damn important for the body to function well.

The essential fatty acids are Omega 6 and Omega 3. Both of these are crucial to our immune system and thus needs to be taken in.

The major source of Omega 6 fatty acids is red meat, maize products and nuts. It should make at least 10 % of your diet. Omega 3's source is sea food. The total fat intake should not be more than 30 % of your diet on a daily basis, while the omega 3 and omega 6 ratio should be 2:1.

2. MICRONUTRIENTS

Vitamins and Minerals:

Both of these are not there for the energy purposes; but are crucial to our body when it comes to metabolism and other important functions.

There are two types of vitamins:

1. **Water Soluble:**
   This includes Vitamin C (citrus fruits) and Vitamin B (meat, poultry, sea food) complex. These vitamins are easily destroyed so we need them on a daily basis to replenish the body stock. Vitamin B complex helps in producing energy and vitamin C is important for strong teeth and proper blood vessels.

2. **Fat Soluble:**
   They need to be consumed with fats. They are vitamins K, E, D and A. They have important functions. For example; Vitamin A is essential for proper vision, vitamin D for the bones and vitamin E to

protect the body from unstable molecules.

Minerals

Minerals like zinc, copper, fluoride, Iodine, Iron, calcium and magnesium are extremely important for our body. They have multiple functions like:

- Zinc helps in clothing the blood
- Iron transports oxygen throughout the body
- Fluoride is important for stronger teeth

The sources of these minerals are milk and dairy products, meat, fish, eggs, etc.

DESIGNING YOUR OWN DIET:

Obviously you need to avoid fatty foods like cheese. But how many exact calories you need on a daily basis can be calculated by this simple formula, it's called the Resting Metabolic Rate:

For women:

$$(10 \times \text{weight in kilograms}) + (6.25 \times \text{height in centimeters}) - (5 \times \text{age}) - 161$$

For men:

$$(10 \times \text{weight in kilograms}) + (6.25 \times \text{height in centimeters}) - (5 \times \text{age}) + 5$$

Now multiply this with an activity you undertake:

- 1.2 – if you don't exercise or move at all;
- 1.375 – light exercise and sports like thrice a week

- 1.55 – moderate exercise or sports 3 to 5 times a week;
- 1.725 – active people who exercise at least 6 times a week;
- 1.9 – heavy physical activities daily

Then follow the simple rule: Do not consume more than what you spend. Some points to remember:

- Have three meals a day
- Drink lots of water
- Have two snacks between three meals
- An ideal diet would be 40% complex carbs, 30% fat and 30% protein.
- Include lots of fruits and veggies in your diet

Visiting fitness fundamentals:

Muscle Building will be the first step when you are exercising for your weight loss program. This basically means toning your muscles aptly. Muscle building burns your fat at a faster rate. Many people have this misconception of exercising to reduce fat only around your belly. No! Either you work your whole body weight, or you don't work at all.

Cardio exercises, in addition to losing fat faster, help you to improve the breathing rate and coordination. While exercising just remember that progression is the key. Warm up your body before you start exercising. Evade overdoing it; like it's not good to carry too heavy weights! And don't forget to take ample of rest. If you don't rest your muscles they may get stressed out and you may not be able to perform much. And there is no best time for exercising. Whenever you feel good, whatever time suits you, just do it.

There is much stuff you can do besides visiting gym. Like take the steps instead of the elevator, walk a couple of kilometers instead of taking a rickshaw, cycle a lot, wash your dishes, wash your floor, etc. And a good amount of sleep is again very necessary to remain on track. If you sleep well, your efficiency increases. Have a fixed time of sleeping. Don't eat before 3 hours of bed and no coffee before 6 hours of sleeping.

Now in order to get permanent results, keep yourself motivated by reading success stories, celebrating your little success, carry a positive attitude etc. Remember this is going to change your life, make you feel good, energized and fit. Don't stop before you win the battle.

FAT LOSS: WHY IS IT IMPORTANT?

Every second person on this planet has one major problem to deal with: Obesity. Following the rat-race many people go to the gym, adopt home remedies and so on, to lose weight. But do they actually know the meaning of obesity? And what is the importance of losing weight? Let us first learn why is it so important to lose weight?

WHAT IS OBESITY?

Obesity can be defined as the complex medical condition of having extra fat in the body, which cannot be controlled by just simple dieting or visiting the gym.

WAYS TO MEASURE OBESITY:

Well, in medical terms, a person is considered as obese when his or her Body Mass Index is 30 or even more. But, the term obesity is far beyond BMI. The need to lose weight does not arise when the BMI crosses the mark 30. There are many other criteria too:

1. **A miscalculated BMI**
    Though rarely, the BMI can get wrongly calculated! After all, it is just a statistical measure, which depends on the height and weight of the body; thus, a matter to think.

2. **The Family Background**
    If at all, the person's family background favors the obesity condition, then he or she should not wait for the BMI to cross 30. Rather a BMI higher than 10 turns out to be a serious warning.

3. **Unequal distribution of fats**
    This situation arises when there is inadequate proportion of fat in the body. Fat belly, heavy arms and legs are the signs of the same. Generally, women have to face this problem after the pregnancy.

Thus, these points need to be considered before taking any final decision regarding the treatment.

WHY TO LOSE WEIGHT?

It is very necessary to lose the weight, because if not done so, the person may develop the following diseases:

- Stroke
- Gallstones
- High Blood Pressure
- Sleep Apnea
- Asthma

THE ECONOMIC PENALTIES FOR EXTRA WEIGHT ARE AS FOLLOWS:

Having extra weight can become a huge constraint in the long run, especially in the financial context. The costs regarding obesity can be too high simply because an obese person cannot work with full energy and concentration. Hence, a decrease in income and wealth may occur.

I think the reasons mentioned above are enough for you to know the harmful impact of excess body weight. Now let us know the main causes of obesity.

WHY DO PEOPLE GAIN EXCESS FAT?

- A diet full of excess calories is seen as the major reason behind this problem. Consuming too much of cakes and pastries and oily food results in obesity. Also, eating more than what is required adds to the problem.
- Lack of physical activity is yet another reason for the people becoming obese. In this materialistic world, the electronic gadgets like the television, the laptop and so on, have made the outdoor activities minimal. Sitting at one place while working will definitely not keep you fit.

IS OBESITY SELF-PERPETUATING?

Obesity breeds obesity. The major reason why people tend to run away from this problem is that the longer the person tends to be obese, the difficult it becomes for him to become fit. But, if you really want to lose weight, then do not try quick methods. It will take time; but it will be worth it. A serious commitment should be shown to become fit, only then can the target be achieved.

MISTAKES THAT PEOPLE MAKE FOR LOSING WEIGHT

- **Checking the weight too often**
  Generally, during the course of exercising and gym, people tend to check their weight multiple number of times. They forget that the body won't lose weight in just a day or two. Patience is important in order to attain the best results.

- **A lot of exercise**
  Initially, with a lot of energy and enthusiasm, people tend to do a lot of workout, which should be avoided. No matter

how much you exercise, the results won't be seen unless the efforts are steady. Therefore, exercise as per the need and also on a regular basis.

- **Crash Dieting**
  All of a sudden, people decide to lose weight and go for a crash dieting course. They will do it perfectly for 3-4 days and then will come back to their original diet; Thus, a very common, and a huge mistake on their part.

It's important to keep these points in mind during your fat loss efforts so that the results can be achieved steadily and remain sustained for a longer duration. Lucy never knew that what she thought to be an easy way to lose weight could be so dangerous for her health. She fell ill more often and developed some complications. Once she understood the ways she was opting for were the most unhealthy ones, she decided to make the changes in her diet and lifestyle right away and emerged a much healthier and slimmer person in just 3 months!

THE RIGHT STEPS TO ACHIEVE THE TARGET!

Well, everyone can easily plan to lose weight; but when it comes to actually doing the workout, the results are the most awaited ones. To achieve quick and best results, there are certain things that should be kept in mind during the course of your exercising.

If you ask any trainer or expert, the first thing they will tell you is to maintain a positive attitude. If you do not maintain a positive attitude, there is not even the slightest chance that you will ever achieve your goals.

WHAT IS THE 'RIGHT ATTITUDE'?

Attitude means the way you look at certain things and situations. As is the case of fat loss, if you have a positive attitude, you can work wonders for yourself. On the other hand, if a wrong attitude is maintained, then you have to forget the dream of leading a happy and healthy life.

DEBUNKING THE MYTHS ABOUT WEIGHT LOSS

1. Starving never helps:
   Starving your body to death via innumerable diets can never get you in shape. There is nothing like the concept of a "miracle diet", which will burn down those extra calories without some serious effort.

2. Do the so-called gurus actually exist?
   Health gurus flashing on your TV screens might have the best intentions to help you initially; but lured with all the money you give them, they surely get derailed of their path somewhere in the midway. They portray that they know

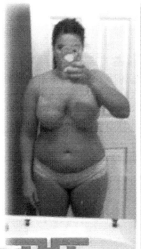
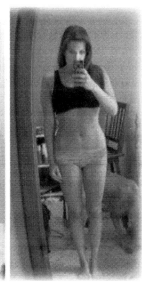
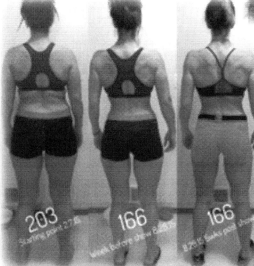

203
Starting point 278

166
week before show 6.2015

166
8.2915 6wks post show

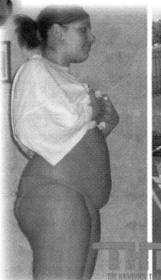
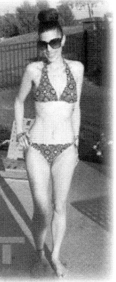

almost everything from health to diet to sports and even politics. Blah! The truth is there are no real life all – knowing gurus.

3. The inside you also matters: While being fit is only considered to be an outside body phenomenon, it is remarkably connected with how you are inside. You have to be strong and wise from inside, only then you can have a beautiful outside. Thus, in the process of losing weight you don't or rather shouldn't change yourself.

4. Being healthy is a way of life: If you really want to be healthy, commitment is the right word which should strike a chord with you. Being healthy is not just visiting a gym for a couple of times. It is rather a very long process. All the small and big decisions you make while engaged in this process will have a larger impact on your life.

Considering that all the myths have been erased from your mind, let's see what actually you gain in this process.

The author says that while working with his clients, he always asks them for their personal motives, that is, what is it that they actually want to achieve. Once he learns that, he works with each one of them and helps them attain their respective goals. He tries to equip us with every inch of knowledge and expertise that is required to hit our targets.

He again mentions that success is not an overnight thing. You need to put your plans into action, if you want to be successful, that is, if you want to be slimmer and healthier.

ALL YOU NEED TO KNOW ABOUT WEIGHT LOSS:

If you really want to get healthier, you should be B.R.A.V.E. There is more to this word than just being courageous. It's used as an acronym here; Beliefs, Realness, Action, Victory and Enjoyment.

BELIEFS:

When you are planning to shed those extra calories, it is pretty important to know why you want to do this in the first place. This 'why' determines your beliefs! For example, if you want to get thin to become more dateable or to fit in your college group or to get a super model figure, then your success would be a short-lived one. But if you want to get thinner to live a healthier and an energized life, your success will remain with you forever.

REALNESS:

It is really important that you get real about your fitness plan. As mentioned earlier, there is no secret of losing weight and it's not an overnight phenomenon. You have to get up and start working.

ACTION:

Once you have done the above two steps, it's time for some real action. Get prepared to put in some real efforts. But again preparation is just the first step. You need to start working, know your body well and chalk out what works for your body and what does not.

VICTORY:

When you see your hardwork finally paying off, you would definitely go frenzy. But one victory doesn't imply that you have won the battle. You have to continue putting in hardwork until you reach your final goal. Once you reach it, your life will be changed on the grounds of how you think and act.

ENJOYMENT:

If you are not enjoying what you are doing, you will finally get trapped into a short-lived success. So it's important to enjoy and learn things at your own pace. Don't follow the universal things, do what suits you and your body. To learn more, *visit us for further information* about the different online and distant programs to stay fit and healthy. And yes…I have seen the most educated men and women taking the wrong steps due to these myths spread by some so-called health gurus! One of my clients, Mr. Franz, a top notch executive, had taken to the wrong way to lose weight. I had a hard time explaining him the facts from the myths. But, once he realized the mistakes he had been doing, he was quick to make a turnaround and adapted a healthy lifestyle.

SOME MORE MYTHS ABOUT WEIGHT LOSS YOU MUST BE AWARE OF

There are many popular myths about weight loss, which may misguide and end one's effort prematurely to lose weight. Educating yourself about the weight loss myths given below is as important as losing the pounds.

- **Workouts mean discomfort**.
  - Not necessarily. You can work your way up from gentle stretches to as strenuous a workout as you are comfortable with. Increasing your heart rate with a brisk walk will do more good than harm and also strengthen the heart muscles.

- **Strenuous workouts are necessary for weight loss.**
  - Not true, you could lose the same amount of calories just by walking. You need to understand that strenuous workouts can help you lose weight quickly; but only as a temporary measure, unless you control your diet at the same time.

- **Activity is not required after weight loss.**
  - Not true. The goal of a weight loss program should be to assist in a smooth transition to a healthy lifestyle. Regular activity along with a proper diet to keep your calorie count within the limits is required to control obesity in the long run.

- **Workouts are not helpful in the short run.**

¤ That is not true. Taking part in a workout program will bring you out from your sedentary lifestyle. Exercise will build your muscles, make them stronger and help you sustain your weight loss goals for a long period of time.

- **I will begin tomorrow.**

  ¤ That may never happen! Consider starting today. Remember the famous proverb: Tomorrow never comes!

- **Working out means I can eat whatever I want.**

  ¤ That is not true. Different foods contain different amounts of calories. Walking a mile will help you lose 100 calories, which is equivalent to eating a cookie. Junk foods like butter cookies and sweetened beverages taken regularly will sabotage your weight loss plan completely. Instead, learn to trade off calories between treats and meals.

SOME MORE POINTS:

- Many consider weight loss in terms of "losing the fat" forgetting about regular physical activity. The two complement each other and are required in order to maintain the weight lost in the long term. Adding exercise to your weight loss regimen helps your overall demeanor making you calmer and more prone to stay put in your program.

- A sedentary lifestyle devoid of activity often relaxes the stomach muscles and so, when coupled with overeating, it places one at a higher risk for illnesses like indigestion and heart disease.

- Lack of any form of exercise can also result in making the body muscles taut. Launching into a full-fledged workout when the body is in poor physical shape can be painful. It is a good idea to loosen up the body muscles with stretching exercises before you begin a workout.

- In order to keep your bodyweight stable over a long period you need to strengthen your body muscles by exercising regularly. Strong muscles make you feel leaner and mentally confident making it an important part of a weight loss program.

SEPARATING THE FACTS AND FICTIONS ABOUT WEIGHT LOSS AND HEALTH

Well, the world is full of fact and fictions. If there lays a fact, then obviously a fiction has its existence! As is the trend, whenever a person is halfway in the process of trying to get rid of obesity, many illusions and myths cross his or her mind, which act as a hurdle in his or her efforts.

Here are some of the common misconceptions that a person keeps in his or her mind, which should be avoided as far as possible to achieve the best results.

- **Drinking tones of water will help reduce weight**
  Many people are of the mindset, that if they rely on 'ONLY WATER' they can lose weight much easily, which is just a myth. If you keep drinking water, without letting go your other unhealthy habits, it will not help you a bit. On the other hand, you will just be found in the loo and this will further lead to a higher consumption of calories. Hence, ignore this false belief and focus on what your expert tells you.

- **Men can lose weight easily in comparison to women**
  Well, this is the most common misconception that usually every second person has. Though, if seen in biological terms, there lies some sort of truth in this myth, this does not mean that women cannot lose weight. If they try hard and with full dedication, they can work wonders. Some extra work and sweating will help them become fit and vigorous.

So just get over this fabrication and start working out ladies!

- **Eat fat, Get fat**
  People are of the viewpoint that if they eat fat-containing products, they will for sure gain fat. This is not the truth. Fat consumption is very essential for a human body, provided the quality is supreme. For example, a diet which is rich in MUFA can help people lose weight, without changing their calorie intake! Thus, an added advantage.

- **Work more, Eat more**
  Though it sounds logical, but unfortunately it is just a myth. According to the health experts, it is important to eat 250 calories less a day and burn 250 calories extra a day, to continuously lose your weight. One should keep in mind that exercising and eating has no direct relation with one another. Do not be under the impression that if you are working more, then you can eat more. If you want to lose weight, just working out is not enough. You must simultaneously reduce tour intake of food if you want to lose weight steadily.

- **Say NO to non-vegetarian food and become fit**
  Well, if you exclude chicken and meat from your diet and switch over to vegetarian

food at once, it is a huge risk. Mostly, people start eating cheese in the vegetarian diet, which is a high-fat containing food. So, being vegetarian does not always means being healthy. A risk factor is always attached to the same.

The above-mentioned myths are followed by a majority of the people. They do not get a proper guidance from anyone and thus, keep following these false beliefs, which lead them to nowhere. Hence, you are advised to take an expert's guidance and do what is actually necessary. Our online and distant programs will offer you an in-depth knowledge of what you must or must not do. *Just click here* to know more!

WAYS THAT HELP TO REDUCE THE OBESITY

- **Stop continuous food cravings**
  Many of us find it next to impossible to control our food cravings. Well, there are many methods that will help you to stop the habit of eating on compulsion! Distract yourself into some other work, think negatively about the food you eat late night or chew a gum which will not let you feel your empty stomach and so on. A strong will-power is all that is needed.

- **Change your eating habits**
  Our eating habits are the deciding factor of what we eat, how much and at what time? If you think that your habits are the cause of your obesity, then you can put an effort to change them, but slowly and gradually. You can make a list of your eating habits and then mark the good and the bad ones, accordingly. Next, analyze what makes you feel tempted to follow those wrong habits and try to delete them from your daily routine.

- **Set easy goals**
  If you start or restart your workout after a long gap, a slow and gradual start is suggested. If you start heavy exercising all of a sudden, it will cause harm to your body rather than making you fit. Also, the morning time is the most preferred time to visit the gym or do yoga.

- **Enjoy your workout**
  If you do not workout with full interest and energy, then no matter how hard you try, the results will never satisfy you. This is because along with the physical presence, the mental satisfaction and interest are also equally important. Try and be fully interested and engaged in whatever you do to reduce your fat.

- **Do not break the routine** This is one of the most important aspects that should be taken into consideration. If you discontinue your exercising, then it will worsen your condition and you will be in more trouble and pain. Do it daily; otherwise do not give it a start. These tips seem too simple. However, a number of women and men have been benefited by following them. I, specifically remember Mrs. Maria, who lost almost 10 pounds in just one month after making these small changes in her routine. She weighed 180 pounds and today, she weighs just 120 pounds. The results came in much quicker.

The above mentioned points are necessary to be kept in mind, before starting your workout mission. Be patient and you will achieve the best results!

THE TIME-TESTED STRATEGIES TO REACH YOUR GOAL OF WEIGHT LOSS

Setting realistic goals is the first step to successful weight loss. The goal of weight loss does not necessarily have to be the one of deprivation. It should be a balanced transition from overeating or complete lack of activity to a prudent mix of both as a move toward a superior life style. The aim of any weight loss program is to burn more calories than you eat. Every weight loss program strives to achieve weight-loss goals by regulating diet and regime of physical activity.

Given the growing obesity of people all over the world, medical associations in many countries have recommended higher levels of physical activity to increase the heart rate thereby strengthening the heart through weight loss programs.

Being able to set goals that are practical is important for those serious about weight loss. When you make an effort to lose weight, it is only fair that you should be able to measure the end result periodically. So the goals should be both definable as well as countable.

- Define your goal as a list of to-dos. For example
  - ¤ I will not sleep after a meal
  - ¤ Every day, I will walk for 15 minutes after a meal
  - ¤ I will walk every day for 30 minutes
- Calorie count is an important factor in a weight loss program. Consulting a professional will help you make a list of
  - ¤ Calories that you can consume every day
  - ¤ Help you measure calories that you can lose every day through different kinds of physical activities like
- Walking for 30 minutes every day

- Using gym apparatus like walkers and bikes
- Setting practical goals.
  - Regularity is the best way to attain your weight loss goals.
  - Goals that blend intimately with your existing lifestyle will help you adjust better with the weight loss program.
  - For example; a program that tells you to climb stairs and walk as a means to increasing your heart rate would be better than those which only ask you to attend their physical activity classes.
- Small steps to achieving your goals.
  - Weight loss achieved smartly through small goals has proved to be far more healthy and lasting. Often those who lose weight quickly gain the pounds back because they tend to revert back to their old lifestyle.
  - Keep a record of your daily calorie intake and loss as this will help you stay in track of the daily goals that you have set for yourself.
- Chronicle your achievements. If you have been able to walk consistently every day for a week for 30 minutes, write that down and give yourself a star. By doing this, you prove to yourself how much you value your weight loss program and are proud to have achieved a goal.

These seemingly simple points can help you go a long way in achieving your weight loss goals and also to maintain your newly gained physique.

FOODS THAT CAN HELP IN ACHIEVING IT

You should never think about losing weight without changing your food habits. Some food habits are a big 'yes' like eating breakfast daily, while some are a major 'no' like eating fried food. But one thing you should accept is that you can't make radical changes in just a day or a week. It is a slow process and therefore, the one who is steady and consistent can only win the race.

- You can start by reviewing your existing food habits like the good and the bad ones. Chuck the bad ones out, one by one! Look deep into what is making you overeat – skipping meals, missing breakfast etc.
- Most of you must be suffering from midnight hunger pangs. And obviously you take in junk to calm your cravings. You really need to distance yourself from this habit. One way you can do this is by thinking negative. Yes, you got that right. Think negative images of you while you eat that food. For instance, think of your favorite pants not fitting you while stuffing in that bag of chips.

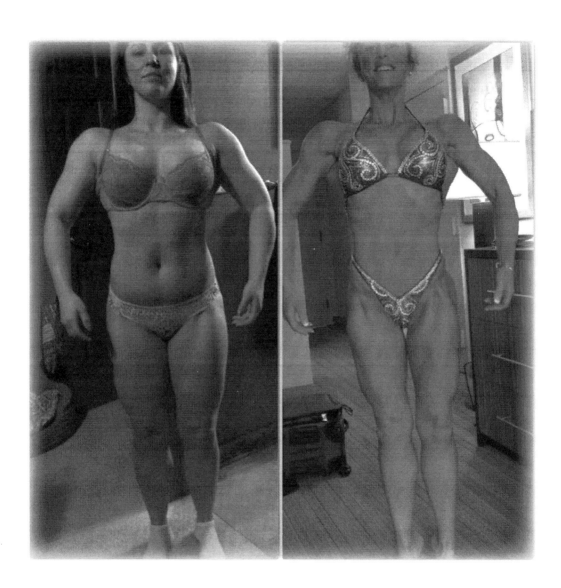

And trust me; you will never have them again!

- Distracting yourself also helps. Many people eat junk because they don't have anything better to do. Well, duh! Do something better than stuffing yourself up with those calories. You can also drink water or take in nuts whenever you have those cravings. Nuts will keep you full for a longer period of time and are not high on calories.

- Next up, we have the intake of a nutritious diet. No one, who'd ever thought of losing weight, could have achieved it without taking a nutritious diet. There are 3 basic principles of a nutritious diet: moderation, balance and variety. Stay away from fad or crash diets as they show you a rosy picture; but that's just half of the story. It is very difficult to follow these diets for a long period and moreover, they don't give a balanced portions to your body.

ARE FOODS LIKE RICE, PASTA AND BREAD FATTENING?

Well, there are innumerable myths regarding the fattening or non-fattening of grains like wheat, rice, barley, oats etc. The grains are bifurcated into: whole grains and refined grains. Foods containing whole grains like brown rice, brown bread, etc. are healthy; while foods containing refined grains are devoid of fiber, rendering them a higher rank on the unhealthy chart.

Eat the rainbow. This simply means that your diet should be full of colorful vegetables and fruits as given below:

Red: This includes stuffs like cherries, onions, strawberries, carrots, watermelon and tomatoes.

Green: Spinach, capsicum, kale, cucumber, grapes, broccoli and cabbage.

Yellow and Orange: Oranges, mangoes, squash, peaches and bananas.

Purple and Blue: Grapes, blueberries, brinjal, plums and purple potatoes.

TIPS TO FOLLOW A NUTRITIOUS DIET:

- Half of your plate should be just fruits and veggies, in every meal.
- Eat in small portions. This helps you in keeping full and avoids hunger pangs.
- Limit the consumption of extra sugar and salt.
- Avoid fried food.
- Drink loads of water.
- Replace those desserts with fresh fruits and nuts.

Mrs. Moody was tired of her workout routine. She was just not able to stick to the workout routine. So, I told her to switch to these healthy foods. This helped her lose weight slowly and steadily, even though she did not work out regularly.

So, a healthy diet leads to a healthy body and a definite weight loss. So get going!

SOME MORE DIETARY TIPS THAT CAN HELP IN ACHIEVING WEIGHT LOSS

The central theme of a good weight loss program is a judicious mix of diet and activity. A good diet helps you maintain the minimum calories required by you to continue with your daily routine while physical activity helps you burn these calories. In a holistic approach to weight loss, one would complement the other without you having to deprive yourself of your favorite things totally.

To lose weight you need to burn more calories than you intake daily. But what is a calorie? A calorie is the measure of energy that is released when food gets digested in the body. Every day you consume different kinds of foods. Each food type contains different amounts of calories that are released at different rates in your body. Foods that are fast burners like sugars and sodas will release energy more quickly and get converted to fat, if not used. Large amounts of fats and sugars in a diet indicate a high calorie diet.

Eating healthy is a way of life that may be cultivated at any age. Adjusting to a healthy diet at an even pace can make it a life-long habit. However, as your aim is weight loss, it is important to eat not only the right kinds of food; but also to make sure that you watch the total calories you intake.

- **Small portions** are a must for weight loss. Doctors recommend using your fist or a cup to measure your food intake. For example, 1 cup or half a cup of cooked whole grains is considered as a suitable amount for a meal. Eating fat-free lean meat is very important and can be accomplished by cutting off all the fatty parts from meat, chicken and fish before cooking.

- **Foods low in calorie** like certain fruits and most vegetables can be used to fill the spaces in a meal plan to smother the hunger pangs. Vegetables being less in calories and high in nutrition should be used as much as possible in a weight loss diet.

- **Stress on eating foods having low sodium content.** Sodium, saturated and *trans* fats and sugars are mostly found in a high calorie food. Diets that contain significant amounts of these types of food will slow down your weight loss program. If these are your favorite foods, then you need to balance your diet by trading off your high calorie dessert with a low calorie meal.

- **Record your diet.** Tracking your food intake will help you manage your diet better. A log will help you manage the transition to nutritious foods having fewer calories. It has been seen that weight watchers who maintain a log of their meals are more successful at losing weight.

- **Representation of all major food groups in a diet.** As a serious weight watcher, you need to continually make sure that you are eating a little from every major food group in the food triangle. Each meal should have carbohydrates, protein and fats in recommended amounts along with vitamins and minerals. If you are a diabetic, make sure that you consult your doctor and a certified dietician about weight loss meal plans.

Following these simple tips will help you achieve your weight loss target in a much smoother way and also help you to maintain your newly gained weight for the lifetime.

WHAT YOU SHOULD NOT DO?

To lose weight, there are some very crucial points that need to be kept in mind. If you are fully determined and dedicated towards your health, you need to follow some very simple rules that will help you in attaining your target.

There are some DON'T'S that should be considered while the weight loss process is in progress.

- **Skipping the Gym**
  If you think that you cannot maintain regularity in visiting the gym, do not join it. Shedding pounds is necessary. But I bet you, it won't ever help you, if you are not continuous. Make it a daily routine; otherwise just do not give it a start.

- **Eat as and when you wish to**
  Many of you must be suffering from mid-night hunger pangs, right? Well, it is not a rare issue any longer. But, if you really want to become fit and fine, you need to avoid such pangs and build the habit to get over them. Distance yourself from this habit and see the results.

- **Impatience**
  A deadly disease, we call it. Being impatient about results for weight loss will not lead you anywhere. You have no choice except to maintain your cool, while you are engaged in the process of losing weight. If you expect the drastic changes all at once, you are surely in some other world. The body needs some time to adapt to the changes and react accordingly. Keep calm and you will definitely see the positive changes in you.

- **Over-exercising**
  Well, to be energetic is good; but excess of something is always bad. Initially, the person tends to act very firmly and many a times, indulges himself or herself in over-exercising. This should be avoided all at once, for instead of giving good end results, it will worsen off your condition. Rather than wasting your time, money and energy on this 'EXTRA' workout, do up to that extent only as told to you by your health instructor.

- **Avoiding the Scale**
  A trainee remains so much busy in his or her training that he or she generally tends to miss the weighing scale. You should never do this. A continuous check must be kept on the weighing scale, because the statistical figures do play an important role in the entire process. This habit of yours will help you to know the exact results and also where you lack and what your best field of work is. Do not miss this at any cost! However, avoid the temptation to check your weight daily. Just keeping a record of it once a week is enough.

The above-mentioned points should be kept in mind, as and when you step out of your house for gym. Give your best and you will get the best. As the saying goes, 'No Pain, No Gain'. Therefore, if you are losing on some of your most favorite habits, you are definitely gaining something that is worth it. In this fast moving world, being fit and vigorous is a pre-requisite to achieving success. Just think on it and act wisely!

SOME MORE DON'TS TO KEEP IN MIND DURING YOUR WEIGHT LOSS JOURNEY

Successful weight loss requires one to avoid the pitfalls that may inadvertently prevent one from completing the program with satisfying results. Educating oneself about the pros and cons of weight loss increases the awareness about these potential problems.

In order to lose weight, you would need to burn more calories than you intake daily. Typically, one pound of fat contains 3500 calories. If you plan on eating 500 calories less every day, you will lose about a pound per week. A maximum of two pounds per week should ideally be lost. If you plan on losing more than two pounds a week, it is necessary to consult a doctor before venturing upon such a drastic weight loss plan.

Following is a list of what not-to-do along with some resources to turn your attention to when faced by these cogs in the wheel.

- **Avoid taking your weight daily** unless specifically told by the doctor to do so.

Taking your weight every day distracts you from your goal of transitioning to a new lifestyle. Instead, take your weight periodically, for example once a week.

- **Skipping meals** will only make you hungrier when you sit down to eat resulting in a bigger meal than you had planned. Start your day with a hearty breakfast. You have not eaten all night and the work day ahead will require you to be active. Try not to wait until lunch to have your first meal of the day, as in most cases, you will end up eating more.

- **Have few small meals.** Instead of three major meals, have five or six tiny meals. If you are hungry before lunch, have a mid-day snack from a variety of health foods available. It is recommended that you eat approximately every 4 hours making sure to keep your total calories within the given limit.

- **Reduce the number of times you do grocery.** If you like stopping by the grocery shop every day, then avoid doing so because the more food you buy; the more will you be cooking and eating. Try to be frugal and make a shopping list of healthy foods and snacks before you hit the store and stick to it.

- **Avoid counting your calories** too many times as this will stress you and you may end up eating more than you had planned. It is a better idea to keep a daily record of the foods you eat. This will help you assess your diet objectively and plan better for your meals.

- **Lesser pitfalls.** There are a number of small things that you can avoid in order to boost your weight loss efforts.
  - Do not taste while cooking especially when every calorie is important to you.
  - Having desert after dinner adds unnecessary calories to your day's diet effort.
  - Avoid foods with *empty calories* like sodas and artificially sweetened juices.
  - Replace sodas and juices with unsweetened drinks and water to remain hydrated.

Miss. Lee was surprised when she learnt she was so careless about her knowledge regarding health. Just one brief session of talk with her was enough to set her habits straight and to avoid the mistakes she was doing. The result? She lost 4 pounds in the next week!

CONCLUSION

A healthy mind is a wealthy mind. In this rat-race of earning money and fame, people generally tend to ignore their health owing to many reasons. Their busy schedule does not allow them to pay much attention to their body and fitness, which is absolutely wrong.

A proper diet should be followed, with a proper routine which includes physical exercise as well. Meditation and yoga can also be thought of, to attain peace of mind and mental satisfaction.

Change your unhealthy habits, slowly and gradually. Avoid eating junk food and prefer the food that is prepared at your home. Though it will be difficult at the initial stage; a bit later, you will find yourself in a more relaxed and comfortable phase of life. The nutrition plays a vital role in the life of a human being. Eat green vegetables, which include a lot of nutritional extent. Do not skip your lunch or dinner or any other meal because of your work or any other reason. It might cause you great harm in future.

Understand the need of the hour and make positive changes in you. Ditch the negative thoughts, which you think are not letting you focus on your target. Do not let yourself feel low or never criticize yourself, just because you do not have six pack abs or a good built. Keep your calm, focus and achieve what you want to.

Just develop the right attitude and you can work wonders. Nothing can beat hard work and dedication. Combine these two and see the consequences with your own eyes. Have faith in yourself and also on the one who is training you. Listen to what he or she says and treat him or her as your guru. Do not take the

process for granted, as being fit is actually a compulsion these days.

Obesity is said to be the house of diseases. Get rid of it as soon as possible; otherwise be ready to face the blunders. No matter how rich you are or how much capable you are, looks of a person will always matter in life. In this much much advanced world, where no one cares about what you are and who you are, the looks is the first criteria to judge anyone. You may agree with me or not, but an obese person can never be considered to be hot and sexy! A bitter truth it is.

Therefore, focus on the issue and give your 100%. Follow the expert's guidance and have patience.

If you have read this well, it is safe to say that you have a genuine interest in weight loss. However an *interest* is not good enough! You must commit yourself to making a permanent change in your life. Taking the first step to get started is right now and right here.

You need to take some time to find a program that will fit your short and long term goals. There exist highly recommended weight loss clinics to assess your requirements and get you started. Remember, there is no magic capsule to make you lose weight safely. You have to diet and exercise as directed by a program to get the expected results.

The cornerstone of weight loss is being able to have the best of both worlds, a diet that smothers cravings along with a schedule of exercises to make you feel rejuvenated.

Never let the fact go off your mind that exercise is an important part of weight loss. Making an effort to find ways to increase your level of physical activity will be rewarding. If you are part of a supervised exercise program, you are well on your way.

You could further your efforts by gently blending exercise into your daily routine in the following ways.

- Climb stairs instead of taking the elevator.
- Walk as much as possible instead of driving.
- Take a bus. The relief from the stress of driving can be very rewarding.
- Stretching periodically if you have a sedentary job

Being *on the move* using your feet as much as possible automatically increases your heart rate and burns those *extra* calories present in your body.

Eating a balanced diet is essential for good health in a weight loss program. Make sure that all the different food groups are properly represented in your diet. A poor diet will make you weak and hungry, leaving you craving for the wrong kinds of food. *Click here to buy the supplements* that will help you get the best nutrition so that you can achieve better health and fitness.

Try not to overtly stress yourself about your weight issue. Maintain a log of all your activities including the food you consume to make yourself accountable. A daily log will track whether you are eating from all the food groups and help root out the high calorie fatty junk foods from your diet. Being in control will motivate you to adjust to the diet and exercises you have to do.

Obesity is a huge problem and there are many well established weigh loss clinics with successful track record. Taking help from such a clinic would get you started on the right path to losing weight. If you are unable to understand anything or find the information conflicting and confusing, consult your doctor.

A problem like obesity should be overcome by setting both short and long term goals. The short term plan should be to periodically assess the progress made. At each juncture, the exercise and diet plan can be fine-tuned to suit the individual lifestyles. The long term goal will be to continue making these adjustments until they become an integral part of your life & style.

Finally, always remember that a natural diet and regular exercise is the key to weight loss. No amount of vitamins, slimming drugs and special foods can substitute natural means to weight loss. So be patient and persevere.

Good luck and all the best to you!

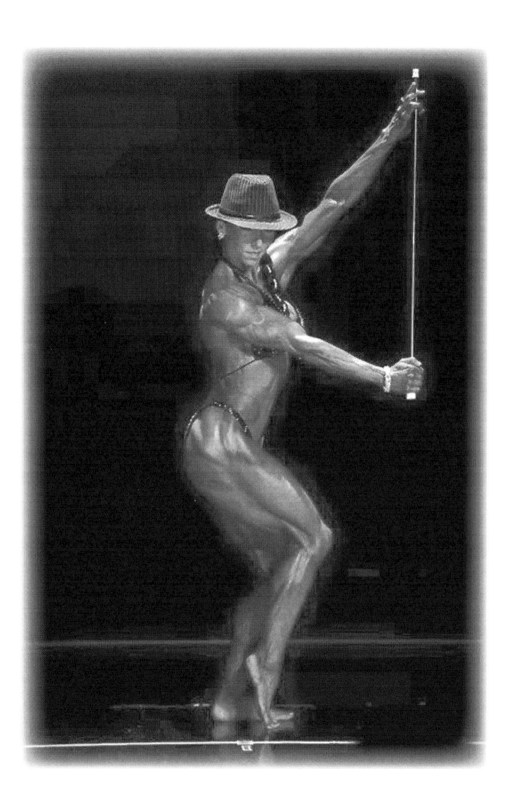

BODY BUILDING: INTRODUCTION

Most people consider body building as a way to achieving shirt-ripping muscles. In reality that is not true. If you have been working out for a while and are not seeing the results, it is because you have not done resistance training. Resistance training (RT) is the cornerstone of the body building exercises.

Undoubtedly, obesity is a major problem. An increasing sedentary lifestyle coupled with poor eating habits has led to its rise. Today, obesity has grown to become a major cause of heart disease along with a plethora of diseases like high blood pressure, diabetes, osteoporosis and arthritis.

The American Heart Association (AHA) has defined resistance training as working with weights to create an opposing force that will require an effort that is greater than a person's physical ability to overcome. The effort required to successfully complete the exercise should increase the heart rate thereby helping to strengthen the heart muscles.

While losing the fat is the aim of most people who workout, there are also those who use the treadmill regularly to keep themselves fit. In either case, you effort to lose weight will increase manifold if you add body building exercises to your workout. Note that you may not be seeking 6-pack abs; but only enough to make your muscles lean and strong.

According to Kelly Davis founder of Mother Fitness, the benefits of working out with weights are manifold for women seeking to remain fit. Weight lifting helps not only to lose body fat; but also to make the body leaner and stronger. Body building exercises boosts the metabolism such that the weight loss continues even after the workout session. The leaner the muscles, the greater are the muscle contractions leading to higher rate of fat burn. This is not possible even with a four hour long cardio session on the treadmill.

Working out in the morning is beneficial as it raises your energy and helps keep your performance at peak all through the work day. Even a minimal workout with barbells will raise the metabolism and keep it elevated for a long period after the training session. The greater the intensity of the workout the longer is the burn of fat calories.

Having more energy implies that you are able to deal with the demands of the day's work load better making the day less stressful. Body building also improves the quality of sleep and at days end you get to have a good night's rest.

Body building helps to prevent osteoporosis or bone decay. Most women are at risk after menopause – resistance training is recommended for building lean muscles for prevention.

Resistance training has been seen to make the heart muscles stronger, reduce blood pressure and prevent diseases like diabetes, obesity, osteoporosis and arthritis. It is neither a panacea nor a cure but a very valuable means of disease prevention.

The benefits of body building are so plentiful that it is imperative for those seeking to lead a healthy and active life-style. A beautiful body that is lean and strong is a great health asset. It makes you confident, lifts your spirit and most of all allows you to continue with your desired level of activity for a long period of time. *Get in touch with us* to develop your body with our distant or online fitness programs!

THE BEST WAY TO ACHIEVE BODY BUILDING

Since the effects of body building can be manifold ranging from weight-loss to tightening of the skeletal muscles, for a lean and fit body, there are many paths to the ideal workout for you. Given this, it is a good idea to write down the exact goals for the work out. This will keep you focused on your own specific require-ments during the workout sessions.

When you work out with weights, the effort required to move the weight should have you gasping for breath such that your heart rate increases and the muscles contract craving for oxygenated blood. The heart has to pump blood faster to meet this demand. Your metabolism has to increase to provide the calories required to do the work. Post workout, the metabolic spike created continues to burn fat calories forcing the body to lose weight. The sheer intensity of the workout will decide to what extent you will burn the calories at rest.

There are many who are unable to separate lean muscles from fatty ones. If there are parts of your body that jiggles, it is a sign of adipose tissues or simply fat. In order to get rid of these fatty tissues you need to add body building exercises to your workout regimen.

Resistance training exercises can be broadly collected into the following groups

- Free weight exercises use your body-weight as resistance and is said to be the most natural form of exercise as they follow the motion of the body. These exercises, not requiring any equipment, are the easiest to workout. If required items found around the house can substitute for weights. Aside of body weight, dumbbells, barbells and cables can be used to create resistance. Mac had excellent results with these exercises and by his own admission; this helped him improve his stamina and endurance.
- Isolation exercises focus on one muscle group at a time. This

type of training that focus on a particular group of muscles at a time will require very intense level of workout for results. Interval training can be used to increase intensity of the workout.

- Weight training uses weights to create tension and muscle contraction.

Once you become cognizant about what is possible, it is better to take guidance from a trained physical fitness instructor to chart out a workout plan to meet your specific needs.

USE THE FOLLOWING GUIDELINE TO COMPLETE SETS OF EXERCISES

- Sets are composed of 4 to 5 exercises aimed at different groups of muscles.
- Repeat each exercise with 5 to 10 seconds rest in between
- Each exercise should take only a few seconds to complete
- Take a longer break once reps are completed, before moving to the next set
- In this way complete the set within the time specified by the instructor.

SOME OF THE MORE POPULAR BODY-BUILDING EXERCISES ARE LISTED HERE TO HELP YOU GET STARTED.

Mr. Smith was looking for ways to impress his girlfriend with a great physique. But, he had never been to a gym. He also needed quick results. But, he was determined to do it and he did it! How? Just read the beginner's program mentioned below and you to will be able to impress your girlfriend with a great physique just like Mr. Smith.

- Squats
  - Body weight squats – with your palms joined behind your head squat and then stand up again mimicking sitting down on a chair – strengthens the quadriceps, glute and hamstring muscles
  - Squats with dumbbell – execute the body weight squats with a dumbbell in each hand. This exercise will strengthen the quadriceps and the muscles of the calves, glutes and hamstring.
- Push ups
  - This is a classic body weight exercise that strengthens the muscles of the chest, shoulder and triceps
- Lunges
  - With a pair of dumbbell – holding a dumbbell in each hand place one foot forward while kneeling with the other foot until the knees touch the ground, then stand upright. Repeat as instructed. This exercise strengthens the muscles of the quadriceps along with those of the calves, glutes and hamstrings.
  - Walking Lunge – Stand straight with hands on your

hips. Place one foot forward, bend the other at the knee almost touching the ground, standup and bring the rear leg forward, now flex the other knee, alternate and move forward. This exercise is good for the quadriceps and the calves, glutes and hamstring muscles. This is a body weight exercise that can be done without any equipment.

- Crunches
  - Reverse crunch – laying flat on the mat raise your legs until the upper leg is perpendicular to the torso, then bend your lower legs to 45 degrees. Then gently roll backwards from the abdomen and roll down again, repeating without momentum. This body weight exercise will strengthen the muscles of the abdomen making them tighter.
- Stretches
  - Chest Stretch – Stand with your feet together and your hand stretched out touching at the palms. Then, fan out your arms making small to 180 degree arcs in a clapping motion. Repeat as required increasing your speed slightly every time – strengthens the chest muscles.

The use of machine apparatus for body building is based on the resistance.

For every force behind a motion, there should be an opposing force. If you push up a weight, then the opposing force pushes the weight down. This allows body building exercises to be balanced.

Such muscles that work in this way by opposing each other are known as *antagonistic pairs*. For example, the biceps and triceps work together as an antagonistic pair to create movement at the elbow joint. The biceps is the prime mover and is known as the *agonist* while the triceps creates an opposing force to control the motion is known as the *antagonist*.

There is a huge range of machines to choose from to workout different muscle groups. They are mostly state of the art with monitors to measure your physical stats like heart rate and fat calories burnt based on your age and body weight.

- Elliptical Trainer
  - This apparatus has handles and foot pedals that you work rhythmically to increase the heart rate and set the intensity of the workout. This machine is for cardio and helps to strengthen the muscles of the quadriceps along with calves, glutes and hamstring.
  - Can be used for warming up for the body building sessions
- Rowing machine
  - This machine is for exercising the arm muscles for strength, by pushing the weight in a rowing motion.

This machine strengthens the lats, biceps, and middle-back muscles.

- Bench Press
  - ☐ This machine makes you pull the weight toward you and release back rhythmically in a controlled way, while sitting down. Doing this exercise strengthens the chest muscles along with the triceps and shoulder.

It is important to cool down post workout in the following ways

- Brisk walk for a few minutes
- Walk on the treadmill

Body building can also be done using Cardio machines, running or jogging to work out using interval training methodology also known as HIIT. This exercise, when done with low to moderate intensities, strengthens the heart and is recommended as advised by one's physician.

There are many well-known cardio machines. For the purpose of body building and weight loss, these workout methods can be selected for performing at moderate to high levels of intensity using interval training for 30 to 40 minutes 2 to 3 times a week.

- Treadmill
- Stair master
- Running
- Brisk Walking
- Jogging

At the end of every workout, take few minutes to cool down with your favorite stretching exercises. The workout has wracked all the muscle groups of your body and you may be sore and tired. At this time flex your limbs, shoulders to ease your areas of soreness. Take in some gentle yoga or simply sit and meditate for a while to relax your body. Body building can get easier when you have an experienced coach to guide you. *Contact us* to know about our different body building programs under the guidance of trained personnel.

FOODS THAT CAN HELP WITH YOUR BODY BUILDING GOALS

You may be exercising a lot, even 4 hours of cardio 3 times every week with no visible results. It is likely that you are not eating right. The basic tenet of eating less than the calories you burn daily is required for weight-loss. Since one pound of fat releases approximately 3500 calories, if you eat 500 fewer calories daily, you *will* lose a pound every week. If you do body building exercises, your weight-loss gains will remain with you for a long time.

So eating the correct and nutritious foods is critical for your body building efforts to get in shape to become a reality. Every day we eat different kinds of foods without giving much thought to their calorie content and contribution towards a balanced meal. If your plan is to get in shape, you need to transition to eating

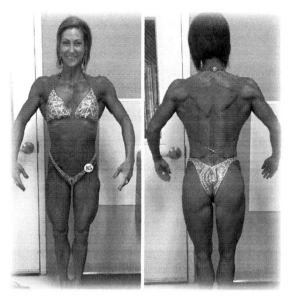

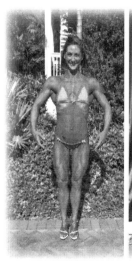
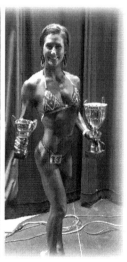
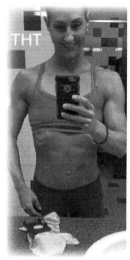
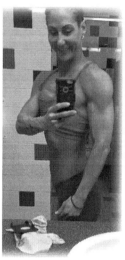

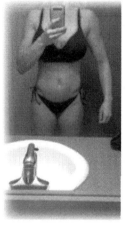
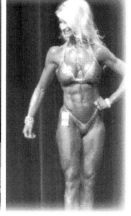

well. This does not mean sacrifices; but only a freedom from foods that will crash your workout.

In order to eat right, you first need to find out what you are eating wrong! So, begin tracking your food intake at the end of each day – armed with a daily log of your meals, you will be able to measure the days total calorie intake. This will help you trade smaller meals in-exchange for a dessert you treated yourself with. A log will make you accountable and help you trade efficiently and build resistance to food high in fat calories.

Put the joy back in eating, share your success stories and pitfalls of eating with friends such that you are not left feeling that you are on a strict diet. Negative feelings may cause a reversal in your eating habits. Instead, consider the change, not as a diet; but as an exercise to inculcate good eating habits that will last a lifetime.

Research has shown that people continually underestimate their total food intake by as much as 30 percent. When you log your calories, you get an idea as to how your calories have been distributed over the various food items. This will guide you to replace fat calories with nutritious low fat foods.

It has been seen that people who log their food intake also tend to lose weight faster unlike those who do not. It is also a good idea to log your meal times, your cravings and the times you were hungry and had to snack. Tracking and adjusting will help you develop a meal plan that is suitable for you. As you focus, you

will find your desires for fatty foods also declining.

Keeping your body hydrated while working out is important as it helps flush your system of impurities. It is recommended that you drink a lot of water daily else you may become dehydrated and feel weak and tired.

Drinking water first before you eat will help you lose weight. A glass of cold water taken before you begin eating will elevate your metabolism to adjust the water temperature to that of your body and help you digest the food you eat better.

As you age, your body loses the ability to regenerate tissue at the same rate as you did early in life. Switching to a healthy lifestyle in early in life will be beneficial as a lean and fit body will slow down the aging process. I told you about Mr. Smith who wanted to impress his girlfriend. Well… I also advised him to make some minor changes in his diet and include the above mentioned foods in his diet. And yes, we know the results!

WHAT YOU SHOULD NOT DO DURING YOUR BODY BUILDING PROGRAM

A brief discussion with Mr. Charles made clear the mistakes he was doing during his workout program. Below is the list of the mistakes that many people like Mr. Charles do. Hope you correct the mistakes just like him and get the desired results! Just read further to know more.

A diet is a very close compliment of body building. When you begin working out, it is necessary for you to go through your pantry and remove all the junk food. Just place them in a large bag and donate. If you do not, they will constantly tempt you and may end up consuming them.

Substitute all your polished grains with whole grains and sweetened beverages with plain water. Make sure to have a tin of protein powder to take care of protein shortage in your meals.

Low fat cooking oil that has less cholesterol causing saturated and unsaturated fats should also be preferred.

Given below is a list of what you should not to do

- Not keep a log of your daily intake
  - When you do not make an effort to keep a log, you really do not get to know the total amount of food you are consuming daily. It maybe true that you are keeping a calorie count in your head; but that will not really help you figure out empty calories in your diet. Body building exercises spike your metabolism to burn calories at rest and while you need to ensure that you are eating enough, you also cannot afford to overeat as you may well be putting back the weight-lost via cardio and anaerobic exercises.

- Sleeping less than 7 1/2 to 8 hours at night
  - Working out with weights requires that you get a good nights sleep
  - Your metabolism continues at rest, you breathe using your heart and lungs
  - The muscles continue to burn fat and you expend calories and lose weight as you sleep.

- Not drinking enough water
  - When you do not drink sufficient water, it is possible that you will reach for a sweetened drink to satisfy your thirst – which will only make you thirstier. This will add unnecessary calories to your meal plans.
  - A well hydrated body works toward purifying your blood and removing all impurities.

- Insufficient protein intake
  - Resistance training requires muscular strength and if you do not have sufficient skeletal muscles, you need to intake proteins to build muscle mass. Protein is available in many varieties. Vary your diet and add the proteins you like such that you have sufficient quantity.

- Not taking sufficient fibers
  - Plenty of fruits and vegetable should be a regular part of the diet.

- Fruits that provide antioxidants is good for the heart
- Vegetables have fiber and help to fill up the empty spots in your meals

- Not writing down your workout goals for tracking
  - If you write down your goals, you will remain focused on achieving the results of your workout at all times. If you get derailed down the fitness line reassessing your goals and adjusting them suitably will help you get back on track simply because you took the precaution of chronicling them.

- Not trying out other forms of exercise
  - While remaining focused is an asset during troubled times; being single minded can be a vulnerability. You must experiment with other forms of exercises, like running or walking, to give yourself a break from body building exercises. Taking regular walks can relieve stress and open your mind to think differently and to alternative possibilities.

- Cheating on your diet
  - Cheating or cravings are a part of any workout regimen. Instead of calling it cheating, account for it by trading for smaller meals and work on finding ways to curb the craving and wean it out.

Sometimes when it takes longer to achieve the results you are expecting from your exercise regimen, you must wonder what is it exactly that you are doing wrong. The solution to the problem may be as simple as not eating rich desserts to slightly more convoluted one as not doing your exercises exactly as required – could be that the weights you are lifting are not heavy enough or that you are taking too long to do each exercise set.

This does not mean that you should give up; but only implies that given your body building exercise schedule, you may need a little more time than others to do them. So instead of giving up, steadily work toward achieving your work out goals.

8 WEEK BEGINNER WORKOUT PROGRAM

Each workout consists of 2 SETS with a total of 8 exercises (4 exercises each SET).

SET 1 is 10 minutes repeating all 4 exercises as many times as you can in the 10 minutes.

SET 2 is 8 minutes repeating all 4 exercising as many times as you can in the 8 minutes.

Complete both SETS then repeat having a 30 – 50 minute break in between. In total 2 rounds of each SET will be complete, therefore 1 workout will have 4 SETS completed.

3 workouts a week; resistance training.

Week 1 & 3 Workout 1 (Monday)
SET 1:
25 High Knees
15 Push ups
10 Squats
26 Lunges (13 each leg)
SET 2:
30 Seconds Low Plank
10 Tricep push ups
15 Crunches
12 Burpees

Week 2 & 4 Workout 1 (Monday)
SET 1:
50 High Knees
20 Squats
50 High Knees
20 Squats
SET 2:
10 Sit ups
20 Side ankle taps
10 bicycle ab crunches
15 Bridges

Week 1 & 3 Workout 2 (Wednesday)
SET 1:
20 Jumping Jacks
10 Sumo Squats
10 Crunches
22 side ankle taps (11 each side)
SET 2:
20 Lunges (10 each leg)
10 burpees
24 reverse lunge knee up (12 each leg)
50 flutter kicks

Week 2 & 4 Workout 2 (Wednesday)
SET 1:
12 burepees
1 minute skipping
12 burpees
20 jumping jacks
SET 2:
20 crunches
20 Ab leg raises (10 each side)
30 Side ankle tow taps
10 Jacks

Week 1 & 3 Workout 3 (Friday)
SET 1:
30 Second skipping
10 Shoulder Taps
30 Seconds High Plank
20 Side Lunges
SET 2:
30 High Knees
30 Butt Kicks
15 Sumo Squats
20 Side Lunges

Week 2 & 4 Workout 3 (Friday)
SET 1:
15 Push ups
15 tricep push ups
20 shoulder taps
45 second low plank
SET 2:
45 second high plank
30 seconds Right Side Plank
30 seconds left side plank
30 Crunches

Week 5 & 7 Workout 1 (Monday)
SET 1:
50 High Knees
15 push ups
20 squats
1 minute skipping
SET 2:
30 jumping jacks
15 sit ups
30 crunches
15 Jacks

Week 6 & 8 Workout 1 (Monday)
SET 1:
30 high knees
15 sumo squats
24 standing side kicks
24 side lunges
SET 2:
30 high knees
30 jumping jacks
20 burpees
10 push ups

Week 5 & 7 Workout 2 (Wednesday)
SET 1:
15 burpees
20 jumping jacks
20 standing side kicks (10 each leg)
20 sumo squats
SET 2:
20 high knees
20 reverse lunge knee ups
20 high knees
20 lunges

Week 6 & 8 Workout 2 (Wednesday)
SET 1:
20 burpees
1 minute low plank
20 burpees
1 minute low plank
SET 2:
100 high knees
20 push ups
15 sumo squats
100 but kicks

Week 5 & 7 Workout 3 (Friday)
SET 1:
24 side lunges
12 squats
50 butt kicks
15 bridges
SET 2:
1 minute high plank
30 second right side plank
30 second left side plank
1 minute low plank

Week 6 & 8 Workout 3 (Friday)
SET 1:
50 jumping jacks
15 sit ups
30 crunches
30 side ankle taps
SET 2:
10 sit ups
100 fluteer kicks
24 reverse lunge knee ups
24 jacks

CONCLUSION

If images of lifting heavy barbells pass through your mind, then again under stand that the spectrum of body building can range from building lean muscles to growing bulky muscle mass. What you want to accomplish depends entirely upon your workout goals.

As you proceed into your workout regimen, understanding the value of different kinds of foods become very important as your diet is an integral part of your workout plan. You have to eat to workout and you have to eat the right kind.

On the days you workout you need to eat a larger portion of proteins and vegetables. Take some starches like pota-toes so that you have enough energy to last the whole workout. On non-workout days, eat a more balanced meal with little or no starch; but portions of whole grain-based carbohydrates to fulfill your requirements.

While nuts are sources of fat, being rich in nutrients and hormones they should be a part of your balanced diet.

In order for your diet to be balanced, it should contain proteins, dairy, carbs, vegetables and nuts and oil in the right proportions. A good rule of thumb is to eat a little from each food group everyday. Variety is the spice of life and the best way to do that is by eating a variety of foods.

If you can do with three major meals every day if it works for you; but if you need more than three meals, add up to three small snacks to stave off the hunger pangs and cravings. You just need to make sure that all portions are small about fist size. It is also a good idea to make sure that you eat at least 2000 calories daily. Skimping on food to eat really small number of calories for fast weight-loss will not help your muscle strengthening efforts. Lean and strong muscles will help you remain fit in the long run.

Also if you are wondering if you have to eat by the clock or should not eat a late dinner, it is not a big issue. Your eating habits should be flexible to accommodate meals at any time. It is more important to eat a balanced diet and smaller portions than stress about *when* you should eat.

Weight training can be very demanding on the body, even when not done at high intensities. You need to monitor your body carefully and make sure it is receiving proper nutrients. If you find there are shortfalls, you can use supplements like protein powder and multivitamins to fill the gaps.

If you need clarification on issues or require peer support just visit one of the body building forums to discuss with others. If you have any doubts related to health and diet always check with your physician before you proceed any further.

BUILDING MUSCLES: INTRODUCTION

Are you looking for ways to improve your physique by developing more muscles while lowering the fat levels? This guide will show you how to build muscles and get an attractive physique. The target audience of this guide includes the people who wish to strengthen their muscles; but are not familiar with the rules and guidelines of muscle building.

There is no shortage of advice and impassioned opinion, when it comes to building muscles. Lack of information is not the actual problem. The main problem lies in too much of wrong information. There is no way to verify what is right and what is wrong. Below is a small selection of facts that you may have come across in the past. Throughout this book, we will examine if any of the claims are true.

1. Increase your calorie intake and fuel up. Read the food labels to know the amount of calories you are consuming per day and double it up. Fitness and nutrition are always interlinked and it is important to establish few rules before you start. To gain significant amount of muscles, you need to include high levels of proteins in your diet. Include a small amount of protein in each meal, as humans have a tendency to digest only the small amounts at a time.

2. Limit cardio and do light jogging on treadmill. To induce muscular hypertrophy, you should start lifting moderately heavy weights. Cardiovascular exercises hinder the ability of your body to gain muscles as well as breaks down the existing ones.

3. Eat often and eat early. A lot of people skip breakfast or lunch. Instead, they should scramble upon some eggs, veggies, beans, nuts, milk or oatmeal topped with blueberries and start the day strong. Eat a muscle-building breakfast and later eat once in every 2-3 hours. Eat even if you are not hungry, especially after a workout session.

Building muscle is one of the important components of a well-organized fitness program. Some people avoid this with the fear of extensive knowledge on how to build muscles. These fears

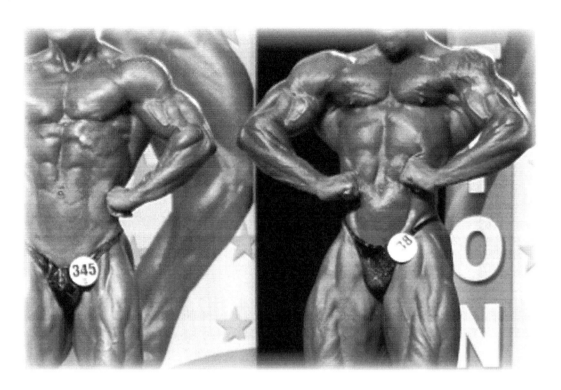

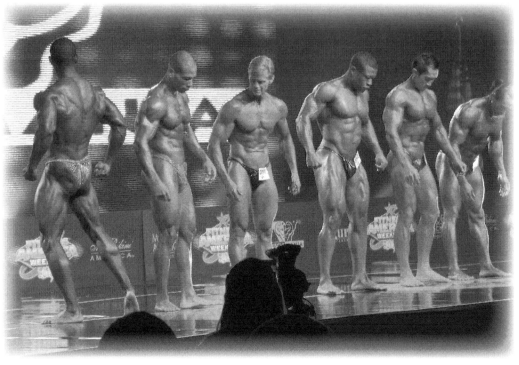

are unnecessary and groundless and it is very easy to create a perfect weightlifting program that strengthens your muscles significantly without acquiring huge size. You just need to understand the principle behind how muscle building can improve your overall health and reduce body fat. Whatever is your goal; muscle building will improve your physique, increase your strength & bone density and help you develop confidence along with an athletic ability.

It is important to understand the concepts discussed in this book before you begin the actual workout program. They will help you choose the appropriate training program that fulfils your muscle development goals. You should also know that there are a number of factors that can influences your muscle growth. You can stay assured that the recommendations provided in this book are not just an opinion of a single person, but are based on the principles of science and will surely give great returns.

Muscle building required a lot of efforts. And for someone like Mr. Paul who had a lean figure, it seemed like a daunting task. But, he followed every trick and tip given to him and finally achieved a dream figure with well-build muscles. Read on the following chapters to learn about the right ways to build muscles.

THE BEST WAYS TO BUILD MUSCLES

If you are looking to add muscles to your frame, you should spend quality time in gyms that will stimulate your muscle growth. You will feel your biceps growing after an intense set of exercises and workout programs. A lot of muscle-building programs are based on the idea of bombing them into submission with lots of exercises, reps and sets. It is very important to maintain the records of your muscle development. A typical routine might involve focusing on Back on Monday, Chest on Tuesday, Biceps on Wednesday, Arms on Thursday and Legs on Friday.

We often hear people saying that they tried everything, but nothing works. This is one of the biggest lies people tell to themselves. They might have tried a couple of things; but not the right things. Below are some of the best ways to build muscles in a right way.

1. MAKE HABIT OF EATING

The best ways to build muscles is to focus on making your meals a habit. Remember that your body is programmed according to your genetic disposition. You should know that the human bodies are programmed to have a good rate of metabolism that burns the calories quickly. So, even if you eat 3 heavy meals, the body will digest and burn those calories quickly. If you want to build muscles, you should focus on having 5-6 meals per day with a gap of 2-3 hours. This provides your body with something to metabolize and build muscles effectively.

2. OPT FOR MASS GAINER

The supplement industry is bashed with a number of mass gainers. If you cannot eat more whole foods, then mass gainer is the best way to build muscles. Mass gainers are available in the form of shakes and juices that are filled with lots of calories. You can even prepare milk shakes at home by loading them with lots of protein.

Health supplements fill the nutritional gaps, especially during the times when you are not getting enough nutrients from your diet. Some of the well-known supplements include – Casein Protein, hey protein Powder, Creatine, Branched-Chain Amino Acids, Glutamine, etc.

3. TRAINING

Gaining muscle mass is one of the frustrating elements of fitness. However, one can gain muscle mass by taking part in a variety of training programs. There are a few basic principles of training that are used in conjunction with another for a significant growth of the new muscle. Contrary to the popular belief, you need not get big in a gym. Instead, it is the response of your body towards the muscle fatigue or damage during workout, which leads to the muscle growth.

4. START EXERCISE WITH BIG MUSCLE GROUPS

According to recent studies, training big muscle groups gives a kick start to the muscle-building process, as a result of which one can gain bigger muscles in less time. One should include big muscle groups at least once in a week and try to focus more on the back, chest and the leg muscles. Change the weights you lift

constantly, as your muscles get used to the heavy weight and do not feel the stress after lifting them once they are trained for the same.

For example – if you are using 100 pounds during first week of training, try to add 10 pounds for the second week. Add some more pounds in the following week. This will ensure that your muscles will not stop growing and don't get complacent.

Building muscles will take lot of time, even if you are doing everything right. By sticking to the above suggestions, you can definitely gain good amount of weight as well as strengthen your muscles.

FOODS THAT CAN HELP BUILD MUSCLES

The food items you choose play a very important role in the development of your muscles. There are hundreds of different foods that can help you build muscles in less time. You need to eat lots of protein, carbs, fruits, veggies and healthy fats. Eating proteins in huge quantities will help you build and maintain the muscles, as it has a higher thermic effect than fats and carbohydrates. Below is the list of top 6 foods that can help you build muscles.

1. EGGS

Eggs were considered to be the artery-clogging foods for many years. However, they returned into the spotlight as a healthy muscle-building food. The cholesterol found in eggs works well on the steroid hormones, while leucine present in them acts as gasoline for your muscle building fire.

2. SALMON

Salmon is considered as a great all-rounder food, when it comes to building muscles. Salmon is loaded with omega fatty-3 acids and proteins, which are the key nutrients in building and repairing the muscle tissues. Salmon can be cooked in a variety of ways. No matter how you cook, you will get a number of health benefits such as – improving memory, reducing cholesterol, etc.

3. ALMONDS

Almonds are considered to provide the best array of nutrients. This nut is perfect for your muscles, as it is full of proteins and fibre. These nuts make you feel full by repairing damaged muscles. They contain lots of healthy fats, which can satisfy your hunger and provide loads of energy. You will get the extra calories that you need without having any impact on your waistline. You can snack nuts and almonds during day, especially if you want to increase your calorie intake.

4. POTATOES

By potatoes, I mean the sweet potatoes. Sweet potatoes are another best choice, as they are abundant in starchy carbohydrates. You can prepare and consume them easily. They are not only rich in carbohydrates; but also in vitamin A, vitamin B and fibre. You can include them in pre-workout and post-workout meal.

5. COTTAGE CHEESE

Cottage cheese is rich in casein, which is a slow digesting dairy protein. The amino acid levels in your blood rise slowly and stay elevated for longer periods. Cottage cheese is also rich in live culture (good bacteria) that help you breakdown and absorb all the essential nutrients.

6. ROTISSERIE CHICKEN

Rotisserie chicken is an emergency food that provides you with the ready-to-eat protein. You can mix it with light or dark meat as per your taste and consume it whenever you want.

In short, you need to eat proteins, fats, fruits and veggies once in every 3 hours along with 2 cups of water with each meal. Don't forget to take ample of carbohydrates after each workout. You will get stronger and meanwhile, also build good looking muscles. Paul was given clear instructions about what you should eat and what he should not. He followed the instructions religiously and this helped me a lot in his muscle-building journey. Today, he makes the head turn with his awesome muscles each time he enters a pub or even a conference room.

WHAT YOU SHOULD AVOID WHILE BUILDING MUSCLES

Building muscles and packing pounds is not an easy task. However, one can achieve the desired body and physique by following some rules and guidelines. It's discouraging to know that a few people are gifted with super athlete genes and build muscles without much effort. Even though it is hard to change what genetics has bestowed upon you, you can still figure out how to develop more mass and muscles. People, who are predisposed to failures, can also rise to the top through dedication and continuous efforts.

In this chapter, you will see the most possible reasons for why you are not building muscles. Most of the guys make one of the below mistakes. You can help yourself from not being one of them by avoiding the below mistakes.

MISTAKE 1 – NOT EATING ENOUGH FOOD

We hear from a lot of people that they eat lots of food, but still cannot gain weight. The truth is you are not eating enough food. Most of the people have a crazy metabolism and they need to have more food than they are eating at present. Muscles need lots of nutrients to grow like carbs, protein and fat. If you don't eat enough food, your body cannot use the calories for growth. You may be able to lift heavy weights; but without excess calories, you will not be able to resist for long. This will have less impact on the muscles. So, it is advised to know how many calories you need and plan your meal accordingly.

MISTAKE 2 – NEGLECTING PROTEIN

Many people don't consume enough protein. Protein plays a very important role in building body mass and it is must to have at least 1.5 grams of protein per pound of body weight. For people who are trying to build muscles, it is essential to include ample of proteins. The more you stress your body, the more nutrition you need. Eating a wide range of amino acids will help you achieve muscle building goals.

MISTAKE 3 – NOT RESTING ENOUGH OR GETTING SUFFICIENT SLEEP

You should know that change doesn't happen until and unless your body gets sufficient rest and sleep. Human Growth Hormone (HGH) is one of the major hormones that is responsible for growth and development of the human body and this hormone is at the highest level when the body is at rest or asleep. There is a great relation between high cortisol levels and lack of sleep. Cortisol is a hormone that can breakdown the muscle tissue and you should avoid it while building muscles.

MISTAKE 4 – FOCUSING MORE ON CARDIO EXERCISES

Cardio exercises burn more calories and will not help you build muscles. It is better to follow the right type of cardio, if you want to lose body fat and build mass. Your first step towards building muscles should be resistance training and not include cardio related exercises.

MISTAKE 5 – NOT SUPPLEMENTING CORRECTLY

There is a misconception that vitamin-rich foods should be taken only when there is a diseased condition or weight loss. But the truth is, people who want to build muscles should make sure that their body gets those nutrients. You can start with a multi-vitamin supplement to get all the nutrients. Switch to fish oil, as it reduces inflammation. Try to grab some protein powder whenever you feel like having some. This will help your body get sufficient amino acids that play a crucial role in repairing and rebuilding muscles.

By eliminating the above 5 mistakes, you can watch your muscles grow and become much stronger. Mr. Prady had been working out for building his muscles since 3 years. But, there were no results. Once, his mistakes were corrected and he was given the right directions, he developed an envious figure within just 6 months!

SOME MYTHS ABOUT BUILDING MUSCLES

There are many unproven muscle building myths that people still believe. We often hear people saying things like "don't eat before going to bed, else you will become fat", "lifting weight often stunts your growth and make you bulk", etc. You must know the truth associated with muscle building and disregard the myths. The myths described in this chapter will help you stay informed about the truth behind muscle building.

MYTH 1 – EATING LARGE AMOUNT OF PROTEIN

Eating an adequate amount of protein is essential for the muscles to grow and

become strong. In general, the amount that is required for the muscles to grow is nowhere nearby. Ideally, it is recommended to have 1.5 GM of protein/kg body weight and one can achieve this easily through a regular diet. In most cases, the person will get adequate amount of protein through the process of protein synthesis. This leads to the growth and development of muscles. There is no need to consume large amounts of protein, as this will result in fat gain.

MYTH 2 – SUPPLEMENTS ARE ENOUGH IN MUSCLE BUILDING

A lot of people believe that they can build muscles with much ease by consuming supplements on a regular basis. There is no such evidence that expensive amino acid supplements are more effective in muscle building than your workouts. It is better to look for an affordable source of protein, rather than buying expensive supplements. You will get a wide range of amino acids from products such as – meat, milk, eggs and soy. In short, the stress should be on the workouts as the use of supplements can only compliment your exercises and cannot work alone if they are not coupled with a regular fitness regimen.

MYTH 3 – CARBOHYDRATES DON'T HELP IN MUSCLE GROWTH

Many athletes think that protein is the key nutrient that is needed to build muscles and carbohydrates are not essential. However, one should know that carbohydrates are the building blocks of muscle growth and act as essential fuel.

Sufficient carbohydrates can enhance the ability to perform strength exercises, as it provides energy to the body. It is advised to take protein before or after muscle training and carbohydrates during muscle training.

MYTH 4 – WORKING ON ONE MUSCLE GROUP

There is a misconception that one needs to work only on some muscle groups, if they want to build muscles. Whatever program you choose, you should keep in mind that you must wrok out all the muscle groups in order to develop a balanced muscular body. It is also important to change the workouts and exercises on a regular basis.

MYTH 5 – LEG EXTENSIONS ARE MUCH SAFER THAN SQUATS

No exercise is harmful, as long as you know what you are doing. Usually, knee joints are controlled by the hamstrings and quadriceps that keep the patella in place. If you are doing squats, you should find yourself leaning much forward. Squats are advanced moves and one should be very cautious while performing squats.

MYTH 6 – YOU CANNOT GET BIGGER, IF YOU ARE NOT GETTING STRONGER.

This is really a myth and there is no truth in it. Gaining strength is often the act of practicing and getting better at a particular exercise. If you are doing the same exercise constantly, the central nervous system of the body may begin to perform better at certain moments. Your muscles will need more fire to move the weight. You can stimulate gains in muscles by improving your muscle connection and get more work done in the same period of time.

MUSCLE BUILDING WORKOUTS 5 DAY SPLIT

DAY 1 CHEST & TRICEPS

Chest

- 1-Incline DB Press SS Pushups
  - 5 sets 10-12 reps
- 2-Vertical Chest Press machine SS Pec Dec
  - 5 sets 10-12 reps
- 3-Incline DB flys SS Cable Crossovers
  - 5 sets 10-12 reps

Triceps

- 1-Reverse grip pushdowns SS Pushdowns
  - 4 sets 10-12 reps
- 2-chair dips (feet up) SS Rope overhead extensions
  - 4 sets 10-12 reps
- 3-DB kickbacks
  - 4 sets 15 reps

ABS

- Hanging leg raises SS weighted cable crunch
  - 6 sets 20 reps

DAY 2 BACK & BICEPS

Back

- 1-Wide pullups Unassisted- as many as you can get out. Then move to assisted
  - ☐ 5 sets - 10 reps
- 2-1 arm DB row SS inverted row on smith
  - ☐ 5 sets 10-12 reps
- 3-Wide bent over row SS Close grip seated row
  - ☐ 5 sets 10-12 reps
- 4-DB pullovers
  - ☐ 5 sets 15 reps

Biceps

- 1-Straight bar curl SS DB hammer curl
  - ☐ 4 Sets 10-12 reps
- 2-Incline DB curl SS Preacher curl
  - ☐ 4 sets 10 -12 reps
- 3-DB concentration curl– heavy weight(use opposite hand to help finish out the reps if needed)
  - ☐ 4 sets 8-10 reps

DAY 3 LEGS

- 1-Squats (Free Bar or Smith Machine)
  - ☐ 6 sets 8-10 reps
- 2-Dropset leg press 8/8/8
  - ☐ 5 sets
- 3-Smith stationary lunges SS DB Plie squats
  - ☐ 5 sets 10-12 Reps

- 4-Stiff legged deads SS glute kickback machine
  - ☐ 5 sets 8-10 reps
- 5-Extensions dropset 8/8/8
  - ☐ 4 sets
- 6-Bench step ups (holding dbs)
  - ☐ 5 sets 10-15 reps
- Calves 2 exercise 4 sets each 15-20 reps

DAY 4 SHOULDERS

- 1-DB Military press
  - ☐ 5 sets 10-12 reps
- 2-DB lateral raise alternate with DB front raise
  - ☐ 5 sets 10-12 reps
- 3-1 arm leaning cable lateral raise SS Upright Cable Row
  - ☐ 5 sets 10-12 reps
- 4-Rear delt high nose pull SS Rear delt machine
  - ☐ 5 Sets 10-12 reps
- 5 –Db rear delt flys
  - ☐ 5 sets 8-10 reps

ABS

- decline situps SS roman chairs 6 set 20 reps

DAY 5: SECOND LEG DAY

- 1-Smith reverse lunges
  - ☐ 5 sets 10-12 reps
- 2-Front squats SS weighted walking lunges
  - ☐ 5 sets 10-12 reps
- 3-Stiff legged deads SS Hack squats
  - ☐ 5 sets 10-12 reps

- 4–Bulgarian split squats
  - ¤ 5 sets 8-10 reps
- 5–Lying leg curl SS extensions
  - ¤ 5 sets 10-12 reps
- Calves 2 exercises 4 sets 20-25 reps

CONCLUSION

When it comes to building muscles, people get frustrated easily. It becomes extremely difficult to build the desired body you want by eating the right foods and doing the right exercises. Adding mass is a slow process and one should be dedicated in achieving their goals. There is no secret to make muscles grow; it just needs commitment and consistency. By challenging the requirements of your body on a regular basis, you can stay assured about the output.

The key to the success of muscle growth is regular exercise and a well-balanced diet. You need to resist the weights that can be handled. Keep in mind that weightlifting workouts are the best way to build muscles. Not only this, you can lose extra pounds and change the shape of your body.

The amount of information on building muscles is increasing on a regular basis; but one should be cautious. If you truly want to change your body, then you should understand that it will be the combined power of all the above said factors that will help you achieve muscle building goals. A solid muscle building program should not take anything more than little imagination and a few hours of time each week.

CARDIO: INTRODUCTION

Today aerobic exercise or cardio is one of the most popular forms of workout. A cardio workout will increase your heart rate and accelerate your metabolism to release energy faster. According to the American Heart Association, *"at least 30 minutes of aerobic activity for 5 days a week"* is recommended for cardio-vascular health.

The fountain of youth is not a myth, it is the sum total of your mental and physical perception of life. Maintenance of our bodies through regular cardio vascular exercises that work toward keeping the heart strong and the muscles tight is necessary to make this myth a reality. The earlier you realize and begin; the better are your chances of leading a healthy life.

If you are even mildly interested in participating in a weight loss program, you should go ahead and find out more about the different ways to go about it. Obesity is a major problem today and in most cases, it affects the heart than any other organ in the body.

Even if you are blessed with an active lifestyle, taking part in a cardio workout program to keep you physically and mentally fit would be rewarding in the long run. A good cardio workout would be beneficial for the following reasons.

- Improves oxygenated blood circulation. Benefits important organs like the heart
- Immunity system in the body receives a boost and prevents diseases
- Lifts your inner spirits making you feel balanced, confident and in control
- Improves your stance, image and concentration
- Eases back pain, sharpens the memory, reduces depression
- Increases your energy levels helping you to perform better

An active life that begins from childhood and is carried on into adulthood will be effective in ways that cannot be repeated enough. Time spent playing sports outdoors and in the playground can be carried on as one grows by an active lifestyle that includes activities like swimming, cycling and walking or even playing amateur sports. As most of these activities may not be easily available, one always has the option to do a cardio workout inside a gymnasium.

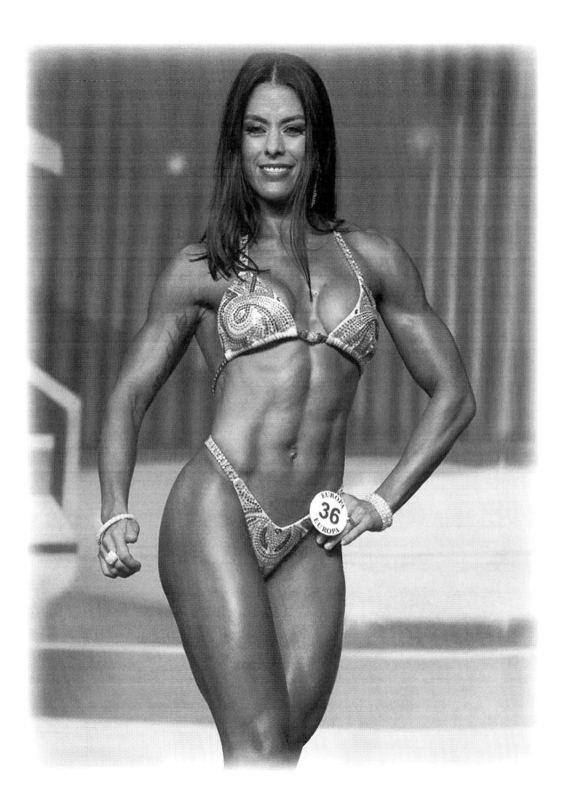

A good gymnasium would have many different types of fitness equipment along with instructors to explain their usefulness in your workout program.

Most modern cardio machines come with a dashboard to display your workout levels, speed and distance traveled and approximate calories burned. Some of the more sophisticated machines can even measure your heart rate and pressure and have an in-built alarms and auto stops to halt the workout.

If going to the gym is not an option, you could still do short cardio workouts in your home for periods of 5 to 10 minutes, at least a few times spread over the day.

Listen to your body when in a cardio workout. There are charts that tell you the safety limits for the heart rate for different age groups that most people ignore. If you are not suffering from any heart disease, your body can cope up with a higher heart rate without any problem. Initially, it may be painful and you may run out of breath easily; but with regular practice, you should be able to increase your workout levels to burn substantial amounts of calories.

While cardio workouts are a good way to be lean and healthy, it needs to be accompanied by a balanced diet to reap the full benefits of the workout. You can burn as much as 10 pounds in 4-weeks. But if you do not eat the right foods, you will put them right back. To avoid such situations, eat right.

Do the math. Each pound of fat releases 3500 calories. Given that you must eat less calories than you burn, you need to eat 500 to 1000 calories less every day to lose between one or two pounds every week. Brisk walking everyday for 30-minutes will help you lose about 750 Lbs.

Cardio workout is recommended for all those seeking to become physically fit very fast. However, cardio has to be complemented by a balanced diet and good eating habits in order for it to be effective. Cardio is the most effective exercise to stay fit especially for the middle aged men. My client, Mr. Cedrick, was extremely pleased with the results. He has been doing cardio since 4 years now. He has become an example of sort for how to stay fit even as you cross your 40s and 50s.

THE MOST EFFECTIVE CARDIO-WORKOUTS

Cardio workouts are exercises performed to increase the heart rate and keep it elevated during the workout. Beginners should start with a 20-minute long intense cardio workout at least three times a week to increase their strength and stamina. The period can be increased to include less intense cardio aerobics exercises as the body gets used to the workout on the days in between.

The AHA recommends cardio workouts that rhythmically move the arms and the legs in steady and repetitive movements, as in brisk walking and cycling. Intense cardio workouts can burn as much as 10 calories per minute and can be effectively used in a weight-loss regimen.

Cardio exercises can be done in many different ways, through yoga, stretches and using gym fitness machines like walkers and cycles. You should enjoy the cardio. If you are uncomfortable at the beginning, bring the intensity down to the levels you are comfortable with, the aim being to build stamina and intensity from this base point gradually until you reach your cardio goals. Try not to *overdo*, intense cardio should be done for short periods to avoid injuries.

Here are the brief details of some of the popular Cardio Exercises.

- High Intensity Interval Training
  - ¤ HIIT can be done for periods of 10 to 20 minutes with separate warm up and slow down periods.
  - ¤ This workout should alternate with at least one rest day in between.
  - ¤ The intense exercise routine tends to burn fat quickly leading to quick weight-loss as the metabolism spike induced by the interval training continues for many hours after the cardio workout.
  - ¤ HIIT is beneficial for the whole body.
- Stair Climbing
  - ¤ If you do not have time to hit the gym, turn this into an awesome outdoor exercise
  - ¤ Find an isolated staircase in an apartment complex exposed to the elements.
  - ¤ Climb as many stairs as you like with gusto. You can slow down a bit if you run out of breadth. Increase the intensity to the required levels as your body gets used to the climbing.
  - ¤ Stair climbing can be challenging given that it has both the distance and elevation just like climbing a hill.
  - ¤ Your leg muscles are on duty. If you climb steadily swinging your arms in harmony, this turns into a great cardio-vascular exercise.
  - ¤ This cardio strengthens the leg muscles.
  - ¤ Lower body becomes stronger.
  - ¤ Heart is strengthened.
- Cycling
  - ¤ Cycling is an enjoyable outdoor exercise that can challenge you in different kinds of terrain.
  - ¤ If you live in the city, you can challenge yourself by cycling to work and back.
  - ¤ There are health risks involved as most cities do not provide a special lane for bikers. Also stress is incurred riding alongside motorized and more powerful vehicles.

However, the health risks from inactivity being far greater, it can be safely said that in comparison, the health risks of biking are far too less.

◻ It is also enjoyable to ride in places where the only other transport on the road is other bikers with similar interest.

◻ Riding a bike where the terrain changes can be challenging and require physically endurance.

◻ Biking has to be done intensely enough to raise the heart beat and convert it to an intense cardio regimen.

◻ This form of exercise is good for strengthening the lower part of the body with not much effect on the upper part.

◻ Cycling strengthens the heart and the lower limbs.

- Swimming
  ◻ If you like the water, swimming *freestyle* with some amount of intensity is acceptable as a moderate cardio workout.

  ◻ A good swimmer can cover the pool length fast enough to burn calories in a 30-minute swimming regimen.

  ◻ Swimming is considered as a cardio-vascular activity that is beneficial to the heart.

◻ It is good for the nervous system and is a stress reliever.

◻ Good for the entire body, as it exercises the limbs, torso and the spine.

◻ Swimming is good for those suffering from breathing problems as it clears out the sinuses and lungs.

- Walking
  ◻ This is the most prolific cardio workout and the easiest one to accomplish.

  ◻ A brisk walk for 30 minutes with elevated heart rates can burn as much as 750 calories. Walk with gusto swinging your arms from side to side in rhythm to do this cardio exercise.

  ◻ Walking is a great outdoor activity that can be done in the park or just around the block.

  ◻ This is a cardio that can also be accomplished using a Walker machine installed in your home.

  ◻ Walk with an even gait and good posture. These are a must for maximizing the effects of this cardio.

  ◻ Try not to slouch as this takes you closer to the ground. The aim is to elongate the spine, sucking in your stomach and stretching your upper body upwards to the sky. Raise your head as you walk and keep looking ahead with your head tilted upward a little to maintain this posture as you walk.

◻ This cardio is a moderate-intensity aerobic exercise and when done daily for at least 30 minutes, it burns almost the same amount of fat as running and swimming.

◻ The effect of walking is said to be holistic for both the mind and the body. Walking improves demeanor and lifts the spirit.

◻ As a cardio-vascular exercise, it is said to strengthen the heart. It can reduce blood pressure, prevent stroke and diseases like diabetes, cancers, and osteoporosis and reduce the effects of arthritis.

● Running/Jogging

◻ When combined with HIIT, running and jogging can transform into intense cardio workouts that can create metabolic spikes for quick weight loss.

◻ This form of exercise is said to be cardio-vascular and increases stamina.

◻ The effects of jogging are beneficial for many types of cancer. Using a treadmill can help patients with lung, colon, prostrate and breast cancer.

◻ Jogging also prevents muscle and bone damage.

◻ As per a Danish study, it has been shown that mild jogging for one to two hours

every week reduces the risk of mortality. However, a word of caution here: jogging needs to be done rhythmically to avoid erratic spikes in heart rate, which can be dangerous.

Mix and match these cardio workouts to blend in with your daily lifestyle. If you are able to do even a few of these aerobic exercises every week, your cardio goals will be fulfilled and you will be all set to enjoy the health lifestyle that you are seeking. Mr. Cedrick regularly performs these cardio workouts. As advised to him, he performs difference exercises each week to avoid boredom. He has achieved great results in just 3–4 months. That's no mean feat for someone who suffers from hypertension!

WHAT YOU SHOULD NOT DO DURING YOUR WORKOUTS

If you are new to cardio exercises or have been doing it for a while, you should get to know some of its dos and don'ts. AHA recommends that cardio is essential to avoid heart diseases, high blood pressure and obesity along with many more valid reasons to have you on the *move* as an initiative to creating a healthier lifestyle. However, many people simply like cardio workouts as a way to release the accumulated stress. There are some dos and don'ts you should consider when doing cardio exercises.

- Do not perform cardio for weight loss without resistance training to build muscles. It has been seen that intense exercising that results in weight loss can waste the muscle mass. Building muscles actually causes metabolic spikes in the body post-workout resulting in higher amounts of weight loss.

- Do not exercise on an empty stomach – it is not recommended. It is better to have at least a small snack before you begin. The results are better and you can jumpstart an intense cardio.

- Do not practice the same cardio routine everyday. Spread the cardio over different types of activities such that all the muscles of the body are used. So, it is a good idea to have a regimen that includes swimming, biking and power yoga.

- Try not to skip your warm up even if you are pressed for time. Allow your body to emerge from inertia through a warm up before proceeding to cardio. A warm up of about 10-minutes will allow the body temperature to rise and the blood flow to the heart and muscles to increase. It will also allow the joints to loosen up thereby preventing an injury.

- Be picky about the equipment you use. Make sure that they are of the best quality. Poor equipment may impede you from working out effectively. For example; good treadmills are not only well-designed to prevent injury; but would also be equipped with a dashboard to monitor and display the speed control, heart rate and the number of calories burnt.

- Do not set unrealistic goals for a workout. It will disturb your rhythm and leave you feeling dissatisfied. It is far more practical to set achievable goals that you can accomplish and will bolster your confidence.

- Do remain hydrated during a workout. Carry a bottle of water and sip during the session so that you are not dehydrated.

- Don't continue with a workout if you are in pain. Stop immediately to prevent possible injuries. If it's a muscle pain, wait for the soreness to subside before you resume exercising.

- Don't stress on counting the calories. Stressing on numbers will distract you from your workout. Instead log in your daily calorie intake and calories lost and review them one a week or a month. If you count calories everyday and weigh yourself daily, you may become disheartened and leave the program. You should plan to review your progress using your daily logs and make yourself accountable for the progress or the lack of it.

It is a good idea to read through the dos and don'ts list in order to know the kind of pitfall one may encounter when doing cardio. Learn from the mistakes of others and apply them to your own to improve your workout.

SOME MYTHS ABOUT EXERCISES AND WORKOUTS

You may be into cardio and enjoying it thoroughly at the end of anther hectic day at work. The familiar sounds of the gym machines or the call of the chirping birds readying to roost in the park beckon to you to run, walk or jog on the moving tread or the beaten path. Cardio is a wonderful way to strengthen the heart and burn the fat; but it may not be the only, perfect solution for weight loss.

There are some myths about cardio that you need to be aware of before you launch into a cardio regimen to lose weight because with too much cardio, you may be losing the wrong kind of weight.

- Cardio workouts are sufficient to lose weight and build the muscle mass. This is a myth. Stressing on intense cardio workouts *will* burn calories; but weight loss will only be of the wrong kind. Weight training and cardio with weights can create metabolic spikes that help burn fat making the workout the correct one for weight loss.

- Intense cardio has to be done at least for an hour for the weight loss to take place. This is not true. Any kind of cardio will burn fat. You can do three, 20-minutes of intense workout every week with one day rest in-between. The metabolic spike created will last for more than 24 hours and burn fatty calories. The American Heart Association recommends brisk walking for 30-minutes daily using the HIIT method to burn fat. Exercise scientist Wayne West recommends that even short sessions of intense 10-minute workout will burn fat.

- Launching into an intense cardio workout on an empty stomach will be more effective. Studies and analysis have shown conflicting results on this. One study shows that working out will cause weight loss whether or not done on an empty stomach, while another says that it will cause the muscles to waste. While it is not well known what exactly happens, it's probably the best policy to start the day with a small snack before you do any heavy lifting. The prudent thing to do would be to eat and then wait for at least an hour before exercising.

- Intense cardio is the only way to burn fat. This is not entirely true as moderate cardio also burns fat. Even if you walk 30-minutes a day briskly. raising your heart rate would result in burning fat and weight loss. An intense cardio would just burn more fat and would result in a greater weight loss in a shorter time.

- Swimming and cycling casually will strengthen and build the leg muscles. This is not true. Only true resistance training will build the muscles. Steep climbing and pushing cycle pedals uphill are some of the ways to do resistance training to strengthen the leg muscles. The treadmill allows the user to increase and decrease the resistance settings to create suitable environments for resistance training to build strong leg muscles.

The reason for cardio should not only be weight-loss; but a means to a more active lifestyle. If you want to lose weight by burning calories through intense cardio workouts, you should take the help of a trained professional to create a workout plan that will be a suitable blend of cardio and muscle training exercises to maximize your weight loss regimen. It's very important to be clear about these myths. In fact, this was the first step in the training for Mr. Cedrick. Once the myths were cleared, the road to success was easier and free from obstacles.

THE 30 MINUTES WORKOUTS

SET 1

- Jumping jack
- Front kicks
- Mountain climbers

SET 2

- Squat thrusts (burpee)
- High knees
- Flying lunges
- Pushups

BEGINNER: perform each exercise for 30 seconds, 30 sec rest between exercises, do each set 1-2 times

INTERMEDIATE: perform each exercise for 30 seconds, 15 sec rest between exercised, do each set 2-3 times

ADVANCED: perform each exercise for 30 seconds, minimal rest between exercises, do each set 3 times.

CONCLUSION

Test your knowledge of cardio by answering the following questions.

1. Cardio is *not* another name for aerobic exercises?
   a. True
   b. False

2. Brisk walking for 30-minutes three or more days a week is a moderate-intensity cardio?
   a. True
   b. False
3. You can lose weight with a combination of intense cardio, resistance training and yoga?
   a. True
   b. False
4. Stair climbing is *not* good for the heart?
   a. True
   b. False
5. Intense cardio does *not* cause metabolic spikes?
   a. True
   b. False
6. Physical activity is anything that makes you move?
   a. True
   b. False
7. Building endurance is *not* an integral part of cardio?
   a. True
   b. False
8. Cardio should be done for at least an hour to lose weight?
   a. True
   b. False
9. Exercise is possible anytime and anywhere?
   a. True
   b. False
10. AHA recommends HIIT style of cardio?
    a. True
    b. False

ANSWERS

1. False, cardio *is* another name for aerobic exercises. Aerobic means 'oxygen'. This type of exercise is done to elevate the heart rate and increase the pumping of the oxygenated blood to the muscles. Running, walking and swimming are good examples of aerobic exercises.
2. True. Walking briskly everyday is recommended by the American Heart Association as a cardio-vascular activity to prevent diseases and as a move toward a healthy lifestyle. When you walk rhythmically swinging your arms from side to side in a brisk walk for at least 30-minutes with a warm up and cool down, it is considered as a moderate cardio.
3. True. This is a recommended combination by AHA. Cardio helps to improve the cardio-vascular system and build stamina. Resistance training helps to strengthen and build the muscle mass. Finally, yoga makes the body flexible, giving you balance and concentration.
4. False. Stair climbing is an effective cardio for strengthening the heart. When you climb stairs at an even pace, the heart rate increases to meet the demands of the physical activity making

it an effective cardio for improving the functions of the heart. Further, the resistance from the slope encountered strengthens the leg muscles and builds the muscle mass. Endurance and stamina grow thereby improving the overall performance and effects of the cardio. This cardio can be done at moderate to intense levels.

5. True. The metabolic spikes happen when weight training is combined with intense cardio. When resistance training is added to cardio the metabolic spikes continue to remain elevated for many hours after the workout.

6. True. People who have a sedentary or a relatively inactive lifestyle should consider being on the *move* in an effort to lower the risk of mortality from cardiac diseases and obesity. Physical activity in all forms contributes to this effort of transitioning towards an active lifestyle.

7. False. Building endurance and stamina is one of the goals of cardio. AHA recommends endurance as one of the goals as it helps to maintain and improve the intensity of workouts that you have chosen to do.

8. Completely false. Cardio can be done for as short a period as 10-minutes. Elevating your heart rate a few times a day has been recommended and proven to keep you fit and lean.

9. True. If you cannot set aside a special time to do cardio, it is a good idea to do it anywhere and at any time. Break up your daily chores into workouts. For example; instead of taking your laundry at one shot upstairs, try taking few at a time so that you climb the stairs many times making it a good workout.

10. True. It has been seen that short intense workouts repeated 2 to 3 times, for example, the 10-minute workouts with intervals (HIIT), are effective ways to do a cardio and maximize its effect on the body.

The idea is to bring a rhythm into your body movements such that you become stronger, leaner and more flexible. Doing a workout without rhythm is *not* recommended as it varies the heart rate and makes it erratic. The workouts should begin with a warm up rising in intensity gradually and maintaining the level required for a period of time before gradually winding down.

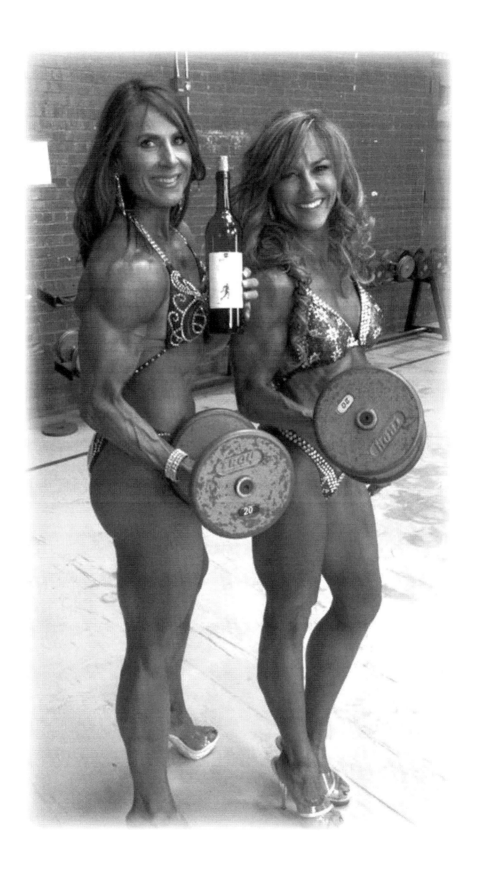

CROSSFIT: INTRODUCTION

If you want to look prettier from outside, you need to start from inside. Well, as is rightly said,' Health is Wealth'. In this modern era people are so much occupied with their responsibilities and tasks, that they hardly pay any attention towards their physical fitness. The thing which should be considered to be the main focus of the life turns out to be the last one. Well, still there are some people who know what their main priority should be. They set their routine in such a manner that exercising is an important part of the day.

Well, must have about the term CrossFit? What does it actually mean? CrossFit is a strength program, where a person is made to do multiple numbers of exercises, without any time gap. The exercises are usually of high intensity and require great power and strength. The main aim of this kind of exercise is to make the person absolutely perfect in various fields; the gym, the athletics, the weightlifting and most importantly, the resistance capacity. Under this program, he or she is made to workout according to the different skills and abilities like power, speed, flexibility, balance and much more. All these areas of focus are very much important in the day-to-day

life. You never know, when the need arises to implement any of them!

Many people confuse this term, as being the name of a particular exercise or workout technique. But, this is not the case. CrossFit is not any particular exercise that you can finish over in 15 minutes and feel relaxed. Rather, it includes many tough physical exercises under it. Burpees, Push Force, Jumps to Drawer, DWT and so on are some of them. Though the name sounds to be very technical, in actual sense you will find them very easy to do.

People should not be so much involved in their hectic schedule that they forget what is important and what is not. The charm of the materialistic things must not come before your physical fitness. Follow such programs, for they really have a positive impact onto your health. You will feel more refreshed and active once you make a routine of your workout daily. Do engage yourselves in other things too, but do not take your health for granted, for once gone, you will never get it the same way!

Each year a new season begins called OPEN. Everyone has an open choice to register under the same and be a part of the five training sessions for five weeks and compete. It is the first pass on the way to the Masters competition at the CrossFit Games. Participate in such events and challenge your physical strength! Only then can you be called a true athlete. CrossFit can be very advantageous to you, if you know how to deal with the same. Do not wait and think again and again over it. Just start off with the process today itself and take the first step towards your well-being and a secured future.

THE BEST WAYS TO ACHIEVE YOUR CROSSFIT GOALS

The fitness models, the body builders and all those people who are the keen gym rats, get bored at one point of time by following the same workout routine and exercising in the same manner each day. Even they require something different, which excites them to work harder. If they continue exercising in the same manner for a very long period of time, they start finding the entire process to be monotonous. To avoid such a situation, the CrossFit offers you a wide range of exercises through which the targets can be achieved. You need to choose according to your will-power and what suits your body the best.

Here are the CrossFit exercises that one may choose to do. Take your decision wisely, for it will have an everlasting impact on your health!

- **King Kong**
Well, it is not at all a complicated scheme; just simple gymnastics and heavy weight. Anyone can do it if they decide to work hard! It is done in 3 rounds at a time and includes one deadlift 455lbs, two muscles ups, three clean 250lbs and four hand stand pushups; very easy to do and at the same time, a very goal-oriented exercise.

- **OPT Repeatability Test**
Well, the athletes consider it the hardest workout. The main focus of this is to test your recover speed and the level of pain that you can afford to suffer. Well, the same is conducted in three rounds after a time gap of twelve minutes each. How much fall off you witness in the second and the third round is how the degree of your recovery speed. A 100% effort is required in this workout; otherwise you may never be able to do it with full perfection!

- **Fran**
One of the most popular and at the same time, the most feared workout is the Fran. Well, be in a standing position and hold a barbell. Squat the barbell at the shoulder level with your palms and elbows extended out. Return to your position while thrusting

out. Well, if you break a three-minute record in this event, you really are a good sportsperson!

The weight of Fran for the men is set to be 95 pounds, while for the women it is 65 pounds.

- **Grace**

  It has a standard weight of 135 pounds for men and 95 pounds for women. Well, the Grace WOD requires coordination, speed as well as your intelligence. Complete it in a minute and become a star, for only the best athletes have managed to do this so far! Give it the best try people!

- **The Double- Under**

  It is one of the most difficult CrossFit exercise to learn. Some learn it all at once, while for others it may take hours or at times, even a day or two. To give it a start, use a jump rope, which is almost equal to the height of your chest and start jumping with both the feet together. For the double-under, jump a bit higher so that the rope goes twice beneath your feet. Once you are thorough with this, there is no trouble for you at a later stage. And trust me; you will enjoy the exercise a lot!

- **Pistol Squats**

  It is an advanced version of the regular squat, except the fact that it is completed on just one leg. Put your entire body weight on the left leg and raise up your right leg in the air. Gently, lower it down, moving your butt back and then down. It is a huge challenge for the hamstrings, calves and quads. Make one thing sure- you do it on both the legs!

- **Front Plank**

  Your palms facing down, place your arms onto the ground. Keep your body in a straight line position and contract your abdominals, while moving your elbows towards the floor. Hold on for 30 seconds or for a minute. Even though, there is no such movement in this exercise, yet it works your abdominals.

- **Lunge**

  Stand straight and then bend forward so that your one knee touches the floor and the other remains backward. Keep in mind that the front knee should always be over the ankle and never track up onto your foot. You can go for side lunges, back lunges, forward lunges whatever you wish to do. It is advisable to change them constantly, for each lunge direction has a good impact on different muscles. Thus, your muscles will really be thankful to you!

- **Burpees**
  Well, this exercise is a calorie killer and almost helps in the movement of every body part. Start of like this, keep your hands onto the ground and jump your feet back in a push up position. Do remember that your chest should touch the desk, only then you are doing it in the right manner. Then, with the help of your hips, bang your feet right at the back and stand up. Quite an interesting and easy exercise! Do give it a try. You will enjoy it for sure!

Well, there are many other CrossFit exercises as well; Sprints, Hand-Stand Push-ups, Handstand Walks, Double Climbers and much more. You will never find yourself short of the types of exercise you want to do. Each kind has its own benefits and way to do. Follow the one which suits your body the best. Keep in mind that what your body needs the most and then take the decision. Do not get stuck on just one exercise for a very long period, otherwise you may lose the interest in it. To continue enjoying the workout keep changing, but keep in mind what your body requires the most. Do it with full dedication and see the results yourself. You yourself will be satisfied by your performance. Thus, start off with it today itself because there is no use sitting and wasting your time.

Mr. Ioannis could achieve the results he had desired for by simply following the tips given here. He boasts of good health, better stamina and higher endurance, thanks to the rigorous training he undergoes regularly for his CrossFit program.

THINGS TO AVOID DURING YOUR CROSSFIT PROGRAM

Well, whenever you start anything new, there are certain dos and don'ts that always come up with it. These do's and don'ts are very important to follow, otherwise the entire effort of yours will turn futile and you will hardly see any good result, even after so much hard work and dedication. Same is the case with the CrossFit as well. There are certain points that need to be kept in mind, before starting a CrossFit program. You need to follow the below mentioned DONTS if you wish to avail all the benefits that you can from the CrossFit.

- **High-Glycemic Carbohydrates**
  Your diet plays a very important role in whatever you do. High- Glycemic foods are the main cause for nutritional health problems. These include rice, bread, potato and son all of which raises the blood sugar in the human body. Thus, not a good thing to consume! Avoid it as far as possible to attain the best results, otherwise be the victim of ill health and an uncertain future as well. The choice is completely yours!

- **Good at every field**
Well, at the initial stage, you will get a feeling that it is very easy for you to carry on with any exercise. But slowly and gradually, you will find that you are good only at little, which is not bad. Nobody can be an expert in every field. Thus, avoid practicing too much and focused only on those areas which you are best with. If you divert your attention to all the areas, you will not be able to give your best. Thus, focus on little and make it your best.

- **Afraid of scaling down**
Do not ever be afraid of scaling down. If you think, that you need anyone's assistance to complete a particular task, then ask for it. If at all, the need arises for extra help or simplified methods to complete an exercise, then just go for it. There is no shame in doing so, because you are just a beginner. Eventually, you will not need anybody to help you out or guide you. But, at the first stage, do not hesitate for it may turn out to be harmful for you later on. Thus, be comfortable in whatever you do.

- **Compromise with your sleeping hours**
Well, no matter whatever is the reason; but you should never ever compromise with your sleeping hours. Your body heals while you are asleep. Sleep for at least 8-9 hours a day to feel refreshed and energized the next morning. If you do not take a proper sleep, you will never be able to learn anything new the next morning. Thus, never give up onto your sleeping hours!

The above-mentioned points should not be considered lightly, for they are the pre-requisites for your better performance during the CrossFit program. You may find them difficult to follow in the beginning, but try and make a habit to follow these. Consider them as your mantra for success and you are halfway done.

CROSSFIT WORKOUTS

EVENT 1
- 100 single Jump Ropes
- 90 Sit Ups
- 80 Walking Lunges
- 70 Dips
- 60 Knees to Elbows

EVENT 2
- 50 Jumping Squats
- 40 Push Ups
- 30 Box Jumps (12")
- 20 Candlesticks
- 1 mile run

CONCLUSION

Have you ever imagined the life of people who are not physically well or the ones who have turned out to be handicapped because of any reason? What would life mean to such people now? Seeing such people, one realizes the value of your life. And whether you agree with me or not, but human health is a major factor that governs our happiness. If you are not physically fit, but have all the fame and money, you can still never be happy.

Many a times, it is seen that people do not concentrate on their health and consider it as a trivial issue. Well, avoid this habit of yours as soon as possible; otherwise the day is not far when you will see yourself lying on the bed.

CrossFit is a way out for the people to keep themselves active and ener-getic. You get a twin advantage from the CrossFit. Firstly, it leads to a positive impact on your health in every manner, as it makes you work out an intense manner, do different exercises, eat a very nutritional and balanced diet and many other reasons. Secondly, you also enjoy the feel of being competitive. The OPEN, which is held every year, pushes you to beat others and take the trophy home. Thus, a spirit of competitiveness is borne amongst you.

Also, it makes you realize the worth of your physical fitness. Once you develop a habit of exercising daily, you cannot go a day without it. You will start to feel incomplete without workout. CrossFit helps you to inculcate such habit in you.

Believe me or not, but a proper health is a pre-requisite to success. Imagine how will you be able to work the entire day if your body does not allow you to do this? It will become very diffi-cult for you to cope with the fast moving world, once you lose control over your fitness and vigor.

Follow the required diet and skip over your unhealthy habits, which act as a constraint in your workout. For example, if you eat too oily food, you will not be able to exercise with full strength. Thus, avoid it. CrossFit demands your time as well as dedication. If you are not consistent with your exercises, you will never achieve the result the way you expect. Also, dedication is required to achieve success in any field. Thus, exercise with full dedication and in a systematic manner. Make a time table a follow it thoroughly and then see the end results. You yourself will be amazed.

Be determined to achieve your target and the success is yours! Never disturb your routine for any reason, for it may cause you harm at a later stage. Work out only up to the extent that your body allows. Over-exercising is also harmful for your health. Thus, pay attention to this issue as well.

The need of the hour is to set your priorities in the right manner; otherwise you may land yourself up in great trouble someday. Avoid regretting in future and take the right step today itself! Good Luck!

POWER LIFTING: INTRODUCTION

Strength training builds muscle by using the resistance of the body to an opposing force from specialized machines. Putting of more than the normal load on the muscles makes them stronger. In the process, bones, which are connected to muscles, are also exercised and strengthened. This may not happen just for the body builders. Every routine daily activity becomes easier with more strength. The performance in all sports improves with a stronger and a fitter body. And you glow with the feeling of satisfaction pervading in a healthy body. With declining age, muscles become weaker. So the strength exercises become more important and necessary than ever.

Power lifting is an intense sport. It involves the ultimate test of physical strength. Power lifters lift more weight than most other athletes. It tests the muscle strength. Power lifters may exceed thrice their body weight in the squat and deadlift and twice their body weight in the bench press.

POWER TRAINING

Power lifting is a strength sport. You get three attempts to lift maximum weights in each of squat, bench press and deadlift styles. You start with the squat, follow it with bench and end with deadlift. The top weight in each style counts for the combined total score. Power lifting competitions are divided into different weight classes to maintain a level field for the competitors.

Power training makes it possible for power lifters to apply their maximal strength in the shortest possible time. This is vital in many sports disciplines. Most athletic activities require fast movements and high power outputs in quick bursts. An athlete may be strong; but may lack explosive power. Power lifting training makes it possible for athletes to achieve explosive power.

SQUAT EXERCISES FULL BODY

The squat exercises the full body. It requires the participation of shoulders, arms, lower and upper back, trunk, the costal muscles and the abdominal muscles in the exercise. In the process, squatting becomes a crucial exercise for strengthening the legs and buttocks and increasing their size.

The bench press exercises the upper body. It requires the participation of the pectoralis major (fan-shaped chest muscles) and the other muscles of the chest, arms and shoulders. A barbell or a

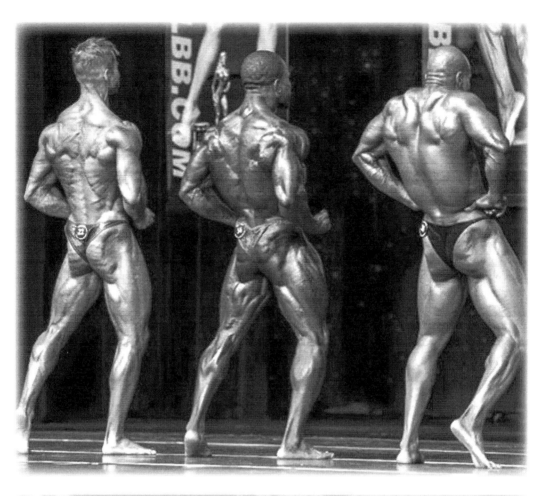

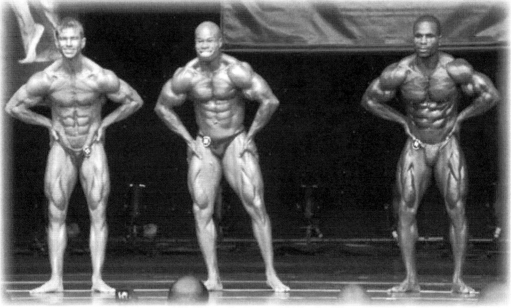

pair of dumbbells holds the weight. The exercise consists of pressing a weight upwards from a supine position. You lie on the back and support a weight with both hands. You extend the arms and push the weight upwards. Then lower the weight to the chest level. This is one rep (repetition) of the bench press.

The deadlift exercises the lower and the upper body. It requires the participation of the muscles of the upper thighs, lower and middle back, hamstrings, buttocks, traps and the chest. It involves lifting loaded barbell off the ground to the hips and lowering it back to the ground.

POWER LIFTING AND WEIGHT LIFTING

The difference between the snatch and the clean and jerk lifts in weightlifting and power lifting is not too great. Both are overhead movements. None of the power lifting movements is directed vertically overhead. The snatch and the clean use the ankles, knees and hips, the same as in the squat and the deadlift. In weightlifting, the lifts are quick. The power lift tempo is slower. Both the disciplines stress on straightening the body. In the bench press, the shoulders and elbows straighten. The wrists have to exert throughout the lift.

Power lifting strengthens the muscles of the legs, back and the upper body. It strengthens every skeletal muscle. The few muscles not exercised are strengthened by other exercises.

THE BEST WAYS TO ACHIEVE POWER LIFTING GOALS

Power lifters usually focus on strength. Good power lifting technique may not always be good for sports training or good physique. In power lifting, the emphasis is always on maximizing strength. If you do not plan to be a competitive power lifter, you can set other goals. If you just wish to get bigger, if you wish to burn fat and if you want to become stronger to play other games; focus on the squat, bench and deadlift.

The squat lift is more useful in building and strengthening the muscles of the hips and buttocks, thighs, hamstrings, and quadriceps. It also contributes to increasing the strength of the bones and ligaments. The squat training helps the formation of enthuses or insertion sites of the tendons. The squat exercises the muscles of the legs and hips better than most of the alternatives.

The squat lift movement starts from the standing position. Weights are used in the hand or as a bar put across the rear deltoid or trapezius muscles in the back. The initial movement, the hips are moved back. Then the knees and hips are bent, the torso is lowered. Then the return movement to the upright position begins.

The hips and knees flex, the ankle dorsiflexes and muscles around it contract, as the body is brought down. The maximal contraction is reached when the body is at the bottom of the movement. During the slow return to the standing position, the muscles contract concentrically. The hips and knees experience extension while the ankle flexes. The heels must remain in contact with the floor all the time when you are performing the squat with weights. Any shifting of the weight towards the toes puts stress on the knee joint. This may lead to inflammation.

BENCH PRESS GOOD FOR THE UPPER BODY

The bench press strengthens the muscles of the upper body. The muscles like the anterior deltoids, coracobrachialis, serratus anterior, trapezii, scapulae fixers and the triceps are exercised during the bench press lift. Pectoralis major, anterior deltoid and coracobrachialis muscles are used during the bench press lift to adduct the shoulder. To extend the elbows, the bench press uses triceps brachii and anconeous. When hand spacing is wide, the emphasis is on the shoulder flexion. This is used to train the pectorals. Narrow hand spacing lays stress on the elbow extension. This is used to train the triceps.

The bench press uses major phasic muscles, tonic or stabilizing muscles like serratus anterior, middle and inferior trapezius; the humeral head stabilizers like rotator cuff muscles and the core muscles like transverse abdominis, multifidus, obliques, quadratus lumborum and erector spinae.

THE DEADLIFT FINISH IS CRUCIAL

The deadlift strengthens the back and legs. At the beginning of deadlift, the weight is on the floor. Pull the bar until you locked the hips and knees. Return the bar to the floor by moving the hips back and then bending the knees. The deadlift is divided into the setup, drive and the lockout.

In setup, the lifter gets into a position that loads the gluteus maximus, biceps femoris, semimembranosus, minimus and semitendinosus eccentrically. The lumbar muscles contract isometrically and stabilize the spine. You stand behind the bar. Hinge at the hips and knees. Set the weight on the heels. Keep the feet flat. The spine must remain straight. Do not let the knees to go beyond the toes.

The drive generates maximum force. You push down the heels, push up and forward with hips, while maintaining the depressed scapula and a long tense spine. The initial lifting of the bar needs a lot of work. Keep the back muscles contracted tightly. Move up and forward at the same time using the hips and legs to lift the bar up and keep oneself erect. Take a deep breath and hold it in.

The finish is crucial. The muscles of the lumbar spine and abdomen have to act together with the glutes. Drive the hips into the bar and get as tall you can. Contract the glutes and shorten the rectus abdominus to finish the movement.

During the lowering of the weight, the steps are performed in the reverse order. Hinge at the hips and knees for bringing the weight down. Lowering the chest towards their knees and keeping the bar close will keep the lift safe.

DEADLIFT, SQUAT, AND BENCH DOMINATE POWER LIFT PROGRAMS

The legs (arms in bench press) move through angles of 180-degree straightness. The sticking points are at a ninety-degree angle for both sports. The sticking point is the place where the muscles cannot overcome the resistance because of a muscle weakness or a difficult position. The muscle lifts the bar and gives it some acceleration. In a weak zone, the bar decelerates. If its speed reaches zero, it stops. This is sticking point. You miss the lift.

So the lifts are divided into an acute angle portion, angles from 90 degrees to final straight angle. In the final extension, the bar speed must be increased continuously to push it all the way. In power lifting, you have to be careful about control and not losing balance in the final phase.

The deadlift, squat and bench have a dominant place in any power lift training program. Most programs will be built around them. But you do need some simple exercises that build the strength base. These are to be done twice or thrice a week for 3-4 sets of 10 reps. Do not use too much of weight. Focus on coordination and execution of the lift. The last and the first rep should be identical.

The bench press will be a good base for the program. Put pressure on the chest, shoulders and triceps. Perform the movements with light weights. Keep the body tight. Dig in the heels in the floor and trap on the bench. Keep the elbows tucked. Military press exercise is done with dumbbells or a barbell. Overhead presses exercise the shoulders and triceps. While standing, flex the abs and glutes and stabilize the body.

OTHER EXERCISES

- Bent-over rows are good for the upper-middle back. They increase the strength of the deadlift. A free-weight exercise also develops the core and lumbar strength.

- Curls are included in the foundational strength exercises. They mean strong biceps, which make for strong pulls.

- Farmer's walk is a fine exercise. Walk with dumbbells —40s, 60s or 100s —in hands. You will improve the grip, arms and even the cardiovascular system.

- Lower body squats will exercise quads, hammies, glutes, your heart, abs and back. You can get much more from deep squats than quarter squats with too much weight.

- Deadlifts increase the muscle mass throughout the body. That will burn more calories leaving you with less fat. It will develop total strength.

- Lunges exercise the hams and quads. They stretch out the hips. Power lifters do not have to move around much. A walking lunge can thus be a healthy movement.

ACTIVATION OF RED-TWITCH MUSCLE FIBERS

In power lifting, body's red-twitch muscle fibers become active. They have explosive power. A high intensity routine stimulates them. The movements may be explosive; but always under control. You do well to exploit the momentum to your advantage during workouts. Muscles have to be under tension for 30 to 60 seconds to activate the muscle fibers and promote their growth. So power lifting workouts must last over an hour. Low reps and shorter workouts may not lead to muscle growth. Beginners should train 3-4 days per week and advance trainers for 4-6 days. They should have low reps on the big lifts that form the core of the routine.

Many men like Mr. Jackson have been benefited from following these tips for power lifting. Mr. Jackson was a regular at the gym and could achieve great results within just 2-3 months once he started the training by following the strategies mentioned here.

essential part of their routine. The extra supplements needed for their workouts are given in measured quantities and are used up routinely.

People also feel that power lifting training will not add to the muscle mass. How can such a thing be possible? If you exert so much and eat the right things, your muscle mass is bound to grow. Those who want high muscle volume may change their training slightly. There is a misconception that power lifters show no growth of arms. After a lot of hard tricep work, pull-ups or pulldowns, a person's arms have to grow.

Then there is a general feeling that the power lifters are slow. The present power lifting coaches add explosive lifts to the training programs. The results are there for anyone to see. They have almost all the explosive skills that athletes in different disciplines have. Power lifting is thus one of the most explosive sports that can be a challenge and also an entertainment.

SOME MYTHS ABOUT POWER LIFTING

There are some myths about various drawbacks in power lifting and its training routine. There is a general impression that power lifters are fat. The idea is farfetched. Power lifters at the top of the game today have excellent diets and their workouts are hard. There are hardly any fat persons among the world class power lifters today. There is no reason why a power lifter should be fat. Optimum nutrition is an

WHAT YOU SHOULD NOT DO WHILE PERFORMING POWER LIFTING WORKOUTS

The squat, bench press and deadlift in power lifting can help you to build muscles and burn fat. Power lifting also strengthens the skeleton. Its benefits are many; but anyone wishing to begin power lifting training should first consult an expert in the field. As you practice various lifts and keep improving your capacity to lift weights, you follow some set procedures; but end up evolving your own style of lifting. You may end up making a few errors in the process. Here is what you must not do while practicing these lifts.

1. Do not half squat during squat training - Some power lifters do not hit the parallel position during training. They can lift more weight, but that will not be allowed in tournaments. To rule out such an error, squat deeper in training.

2. Do not ignore the pause at the chest in bench pressing training. This may reduce your loads by about 10 percent in the short run. But ultimately you will emerge stronger and lift more. Pause longer at the chest during practice so that you can perform better at official meets.

3. Do not ignore optimal warming up. A ten-minute warming up period is usually good. Do not lift high weights during the warming up period.

4. Do not shun experimenting with training gear. Try various types of gears during the training period. You have to use various types of gear to find out which suits you the best. Try different shoes, knee wraps, belts and singlets.

5. Do not ruin your peaking process. Take it easy for a few days before a special meet. Do not lift during this period. Do not change your normal foods. Do not try anything suddenly.

6. Do not fail to film your lifts. Ensure that you are squatting well below the right level during practice. Watch the videos, ensure that your pause is proper and all your lifts are correct.

7. Do not be without a training partner or a coach. They point out mistakes, tell you that you have not practiced enough and they also give good advice. But do not over-rely on the coach. You have to have your own plan too.

8. Do not forget to bring your own supplies. You are used to some supplies and gears. If these are changed, your performance could be affected badly.

9. Avoid extra wide stances and grips. It may seem easier to reach the parallel squat with an extra wide stance; but it will irritate the hip joints and lead to a loss of smooth motion. An ultra-wide grip may cut down the motion of the bench press; but will put burden on the shoulders and reduce triceps contribution.

10. Do not overarch the back in the bench press. Such tense spine reduces the range of motion.

11. Do not tuck the elbows too much. They prevent the elbows from staying under the wrists, thus burdening the shoulders.

12. Avoid very low reps. Using moderate reps and heavier weights will be safer.

13. Avoid speed work. Fast movement exercise fast-twitch muscle fibers, but not well enough. Slower movements make possible more connections to form. You still need a high effort to use the fast-twitch muscle fibers.

14. Avoid too many warm-up sets. This serves no purpose. It will exhaust you quite early. Go for just one or two warm-up sets. Save energy for the real battle.

15. Avoid power lifting for general training.

16. Avoid deadlifting. Deadlifting with a barbell lays stress on the hip extensors and the lower back, ignoring the quads and calves. It may also harm the spine and hips.

POWERLIFTING 5 DAY WORKOUTS

DAY 1 CHEST /TRICEP

- Flat Bench Chest Press
  - ¤ 5 sets 10-12 reps
- Incline DB Press
  - ¤ 5 sets 10-12 reps

- Machine Flys or DB Flys or Pec Dec Machine
  - ¤ 5 sets 10-12 reps
- Reverse grip pushdowns SS Pushdowns
  - ¤ 4 sets 10-12 reps
- Skull Crushers w EZ Bar
  - ¤ 4 sets 10-12 reps
- Rope overhead extensions
  - ¤ 4 sets 10-12 reps

DAY 2 SHOULDERS & ABS

- Machine OH Press
  - ¤ 5 sets 6-10 reps
- Cable lateral raise
  - ¤ 5 sets 10-12 reps
- DB 1 Arm Front Raise
  - ¤ 5 sets 6-10 reps
- Rear Delt Reverse Flys w Cable or DB
  - ¤ 5 sets 10-12 reps
- Db upright row
  - ¤ 5 sets 8-10 reps
- Machine Crunches
  - ¤ 4 Sets of 20
- Planks
  - ¤ 30 Secs Holds

DAY 3 BACK/BICEPS

- Straight bar curl w EZ Bar
  - ¤ 4 sets 10-12 reps
- Incline DB curl
  - ¤ 4 sets 10-12 reps
- Hammer Curls w DB
  - ¤ 3 sets of 15
- Wide pullups Assisted
  - ¤ 5 sets to Failure

- 1 arm DB row
  - ¤ 5 sets 10-12 reps
- Close grip seated row
  - ¤ 5 sets 10-12 reps

DAY 4 LEGS

- Machine Press
  - ¤ 6 sets 10-12 reps
- Leg Extension
  - ¤ 5 sets 12-15 Reps
- Smith stationary lunges
  - ¤ 5 sets 10-12 Reps
- Lying Leg Curls
  - ¤ 5 sets 8-10 reps
- Calf Raise Machine
  - ¤ 4 sets of 10

CONCLUSION

Power lifting is a game of strength. You perform reps of the squat, bench press and deadlift regularly to lift more weight, gain strength, lose weight and to look muscular and better. It is popular among fitness enthusiasts. In power lifting, safety is of utmost importance. The main tool to ensure safety is to learn and master the correct technique in each of the lift exercises. Your technique has to be perfect. The coach should watch all your moves all the time, especially during your initial learning phase and keep correcting each minor flaw to leave you with a faultless technique. Any slightest flaw in the technique can land you in trouble, especially when lifting heavy weights.

Right equipment a vital factor

The power lifters need the right equipment. For squats, a squat rack equipped with adjustable safety bars is a necessity. You need a training partner for keeping a watch during bench pressing. You must not be trapped under the bar.

Whatever be the purpose of power lifting routine, you can do better by following these procedures regularly.

1. Before beginning to lift heavy weights, you must get fully used to the technique of each of the lifts. The process must become automatic for your body. Practice the lifts continuously until you master the technique. Thousands of reps will make your lift flawless and will raise your strength. That is the moment for you to start lifting higher and higher weights.

2. Be focused. Ensure that you focus on the three core lifts of the squat, bench press and the deadlift and stay with them until you master them. Only then you can think of other lifts. Concentrate on the basics in the early stages.

3. Seek help. The various power lifts can be quite confusing. Many alternative movements can occur to you. There are innumerable equipment, training programs and techniques available. You cannot decide which to select. You do not know what to eat or what supplements are required. So it is better to find an experienced coach and profit by his/ her advice.

4. Search of the right gym. The gym you train in is important for power lifters. A beginner can get some advice too in the right gym. Many gyms have equipment necessary for a specific lift. This can be an added advantage.

5. Watch and learn. You can learn a lot by watching others perform. Get acquainted with the basics by watching competitions. You can also see how the competitors prepare themselves mentally and how they warm up for each lift.

6. Good equipment. You achieve the best results if you acquire the best technique and use the best gear. Make sure that the singlets, straps, sleeves, compression garments and belts meet the standards laid down by the tournament organizers and are approved by them.

7. Protect your hands. As you work harder, calluses will form on palms where you grip the bar. Use a stone to wear these calluses down and keep the hands in good condition. Do not try to tear down the calluses.

8. Be slow but steady. You cannot expect to lift huge within months. It takes time to build strength. Evolve comfortable training program. Enjoy it. Set goals for distant dates. Be happy with every small achievement. Do not be disheartened if the progress is slow.

9. Have a clean lifestyle. Decide for yourself if your present lifestyle is conducive to power lifting. Change it if that is necessary. Unless you are committed to the idea, you will not be able to do much in power lifting.

10. If you plan to participate in power lifting tournaments, get familiar with the commands issued by the referee. You have to know all the rules governing the contest. You have to have a ready strategy for the competition. You should know your opening weights and how you are going to increase them. You should not over-exercise during the warming up period.

Good Luck!!!

STRENGTH TRAINING: INTRODUCTION

Good job, you have decided to get fit! You are now about to enter into a world where all your physical and mental faculties will be challenged. A lot of patience and dedication will be needed from you to stay with the workout program. This is a brief guide on strength training.

If you have done aerobic exercises in the past and are wondering what additional benefits strength training has to offer, then you need to understand the basic differences between cardio and weight training. In the world of exercise, there are two terms you need to comprehend, one is aerobic, which means with air and the other anaerobic, which means without air. Aerobic exercises build endurance and stamina while anaerobic exercises build strength.

Aerobic exercises increase you heart rate to the levels high enough to burn carbohydrate and fats. It makes the heart work hard to pump oxygenated blood throughout the system and is known as a *cardio workout*.

Anaerobic exercises use weights to create muscular contractions. This helps to build muscles and keeps the metabolism elevated for a long time allowing the body to burn calories even at rest. *Weight training* is an example.

According to a scientific statement made by a group of physicians affiliated to the American Heart Association (AHA), a supervised resistance training *"increases muscular strength and also the quality of life while reducing the disability in people with or without any cardio-vascular disease."*

Our heart and lungs are very important organs and every day, we involuntarily expose them to unhealthy pollutants like second hand smoke. It is imperative that we learn to treat them well through regular cardio activity. The AHA, concerned with growing obesity amongst adults as the main cause behind the increase in the incidence of heart disease, have recommended anaerobic cardio-vascular activity like brisk walking with small intervals of rest to stimulate the heart rate and make the heart muscles stronger. You may get in touch with us to *buy the supplements* that will provide you best nutrition and help you achieve better health and fitness.

The effect of aerobic exercises is increased endurance, weight-loss and improved cardio-vascular functioning of the heart. However, this does not lead to lean body mass. The muscles grow

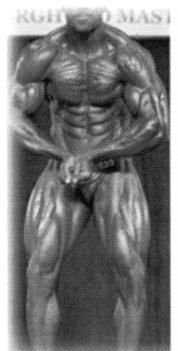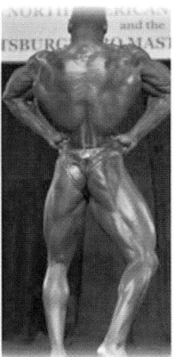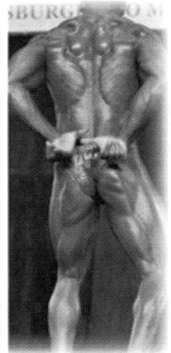
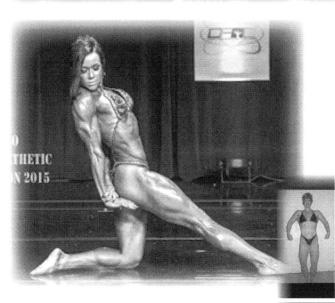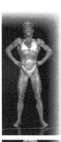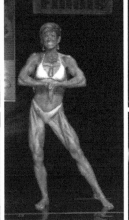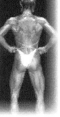

stronger; but not as much as with the anaerobic exercises.

It is resistance or weight training that causes weight-loss through increased metabolism. Intense anaerobic activity like lifting heavy weights that leave you gasping for breath cause metabolic spikes that help you burn fat for long periods after the workout session. The resulting *burn* of adipose tissues leads to a lean body mass.

Quality of life is very important as it enables you to do the things you want every day. Any impediment, like disease or illness, can affect your ability to perform your daily tasks. Even in these extreme circumstances, you can do anaerobic exercises to rehabilitate your life.

The *daily burn* is not the name of a newspaper, but an eagerly sought-after energy release of fat calories through metabolic exercises. Anaerobic exercises performed 2 to 3 times a week for 20–50 minutes will help you build muscle mass and make you stronger.

The cornerstone of metabolic exercise is resistance training (RT) using weights. Supervised RT has been recommended by AHA for the prevention of chronic diseases like cardio-vascular, high blood pressure, obesity, diabetes and for weight-loss management.

If your concern is with weight-loss; the good news is that growing muscle mass with the help of anaerobic exercises like RT can help to sustain the weight loss gained for a longer time.

Now that you know what strength training is; you can proceed to create a workout schedule suitable for your needs.

THE BEST WAYS TO ACHIEVE YOUR STRENGTH TRAINING GOALS

Strength training is exercising with weights. Lifting, pulling and pushing weights such that you build muscle mass by resisting to forces that are greater than your body mass. The heavier the weights; the more intense is the exercise.

Your aim for resistance training (RT) is to work against an opposing force that is greater than your own physical strength. The effort made by you should have you out of breath within a few minutes. When repeated a few times with intervals of rest, the effort will build lean muscle mass and make your skeletal muscles strong.

In weight training, you can use your own body as resistance. As these exercises do not need weights, you can do them anywhere, without having to go to a gym. A few of them that do require a weight, items found around the house can be substituted.

The following types of exercises are the most basic for building strength in the different muscle groups.

- Push – these exercises are good for the pectoral, shoulder and triceps. The abdominal and back muscles are used to hold the form of the body while doing the above exercises.
  - ◻ Mountain Climber – the individual resumes a classic push-up position and then

brings up the left knee to the chest, hops to straighten the left knee and bring up the right knee.

◻ Helps to strengthen the shoulder, abdominals and core muscles

● Push-ups – Strengthens all the skeletal muscles and is a popular form of exercise.

◻ This exercise builds the pectoral, triceps and deltoids.

● Pull – Exercises use resistive-pulling motion to build different muscle-groups.

◊ Pull up is a well-known exercise where a bar is used to pull one up and lower oneself again with the general form held upright and in a hanging position from the bar.

◊ The deltoids, spine, biceps and abdominal muscles are strengthened by these exercises.

● Core – This form of exercising is directed at the back and abdominal muscles.

◻ Crunch is a popular exercise for the tightening of abdominal muscles.

◊ This exercise requires lying on the floor with hands behind the head and raising the upper back while keeping the lower back flat on the ground.

◻ Flutter Kicks – This is done by lying on the ground and raising both legs up together slightly from the ground.

Then raise one leg at a time to 45 degrees and down again.

● Legs/Glutes – The thigh, calf and glute muscles are strengthened by these exercises. Some of the popular exercises are

◻ Squat jumps to build lower body strength

◻ Dead lifts will strengthen the hamstrings and lower back

The only problem with body weight exercises is that the resistance never exceeds one's own weight. This means that the intensity of the exercises will never be close to the maximum weight that one may be able to lift. A weighted-suit can be used to increase the body weight; but then that will again take one to the gym or a store to purchase equipment. Some additional ways to do bodyweight training that will affect all the muscle groups is by running uphill, treadmills, skipping and jogging.

Weight training undoubtedly requires guidance from a certified instructor, who will help you get started on the right foot. For inexperienced beginners, it is recommended that they begin their workouts with machines. The body is not trained to lift weights and injuries can happen. Starting out on machines will help you workout the entire or specific muscles groups as required and condition them for free weight exercises.

The general instructions for using machines are

- Workout 2 to 3 times a week
- Repeat each exercise 8-12 times
- Maximum of 5-seconds to do a single repetition
- Exercise each set until you are fatigued, then rest
- Take between 1 and 1½ minutes rest in between

The following are some of the machines that you can use for weight training

- Cardio Warm up for 10-minutes
  - Treadmill – for walking, jogging and running using flat or uphill terrain
  - Your heart rate will increase and your circulation will improve causing a better flow of oxygenated blood all through your system.
- Weights workout in 20-50 minute sessions
  - Leg press will strengthen your ankle muscles and all the muscles of your legs and lower body
  - Leg Extensions will work to strengthen the leg muscles called quadriceps
  - Lying/Seated leg curls will strengthen your hamstrings
  - Lat Pull down will strengthen the shoulders, back muscles and biceps
  - Bench Press Machine will strengthen the muscles of the chest, shoulders and triceps
  - Ab Crunch machine will help strengthen the abdominal muscles

It has been argued that working out specific areas of the body does not work as muscle strengthening. It depends on the body composition. The latter decides in which order the different muscle groups will be strengthened. So, it is a good idea to work on a few muscle groups at a time and not any single one when you work out.

Make weight training a light-hearted exercise by sharing your experiences with others. Share your success stories, photographs and the training faux-pas with friends and peers to keep your training going smoothly as well as staying informed and educated.

FOODS THAT CAN HELP IN YOUR STRENGTH TRAINING PROGRAM

While weight training takes care of your muscles, you also need to eat the right kinds of foods to make the training successful. Whether you aim is to gain weight-loss or general fitness, you have a good chance of crashing out of your program when you eat the wrong kind of foods.

The general rule of the thumb is to eat a balanced meal with all the food groups represented in your diet. Sometimes a metabolic diet is used to complement anaerobic exercises for fast results. However, due to the controversial nature of these diets, they are not recommended. If you choose to use these diets, talk to an expert first and get his approval.

The goal of your exercise regimen should be physical fitness. For good health and to get the vitality and energy to carry on your daily activities, you need to eat from the three major food groups: carbohydrates, proteins and fats. The best diet for weight-loss has been proven to be ones with large amounts of proteins and dairy. A diet that contains up to 30% proteins and dairy is recommended for weight loss. If the goal is building muscle mass, then a fat-free starchy diet is recommended.

Listed here are some of the foods in each major food group that can be used in diet plans to build muscle mass when accompanied by weight training.

- Carbohydrates or starches
  - Whole grains, unpolished rice, starches like yams and potatoes
- Proteins
  - White meats and fish, eggs, dairy and legumes
- Fruits and Vegetables
  - Citrus fruits and all vegetables
- Fats and oils
  - As little as possible

The diet should provide at least 2500 calories per day with equal amounts of carbohydrates and proteins and a small quantity of fat. Some starches burn faster than others. For example: rice, breads and pasta are considered to be the foods high in starch; while fruits and whole grains contain fiber and are considered less starchy. So, they take more time to burn the calories.

The presence of starch in the diet helps fuel the increase in the rate of metabolism required for weight training.

Some healthy eating habits to build strong muscles

- To grow lean muscles, you have to eat to maintain your metabolism
- Pay attention to the hydration needs of your body. Avoid sweetened drinks and drink plenty of water
- Replace all polished grains with whole grains and unpolished rice
- Eat a small snack before workout.
- Eat plenty of fruits and vegetables and only lean meats
- To prevent cravings, eat 5 to 6 meals daily: Three major meals and 2 to 3 small ones in between.
- Add a teaspoon of protein powder to your smoothie if you fall short of the required protein intake.

Knowing about the types of foods and their values to your strength training effort will help you put together your meal plans that are balanced.

If you are on a weight-loss regimen, a workout on an empty stomach is alright before breakfast. But, if your goal is to workout intensely for building muscles, taking a small snack pre-workout will help you.

- For improved performance, eat a healthy snack within 200 calories, 30-minutes before workout to have a good energy level.

You must also know *when* to eat. According to some experts *"timing is everything!"*

- Do not eat both before and after a workout.
- Eat within 30-minutes of finishing a workout to help the muscles recover.
- Time your workout to end such that they coincide with major meals.
- Foods high on antioxidants like cherry juices help in muscle recovery.

Strength training requires you to take lots more protein. If you are unsure, track your food intake and discuss it with your instructor. Keeping a small stash of healthy snacks within reach will help stop the cravings as well as keep you on track for eating nutritiously.

THINGS TO AVOID DURING YOUR STRENGTH TRAINING PROGRAM

There are plenty of dos and don'ts as the opinions differ between instructors. When in doubt, the best thing to do is to consult a physician.

- Weight training with large weights.
  - Work your way up from small weights to heavier ones within your ability. Control will help you to execute the exercise correctly.
  - Having high expectations and starting with too much weight can make you falter and may put you at a risk for injury. Tired and disillusioned, you may even leave the program.
- Training with too little weight
  - It is recommended that if you can repeat an exercise with the given weight, consider raising the weight.
  - Raising the weights 5% at a time ensures that you are not hassled and are able to make a smooth transition to larger weights while keeping yourself safe from injuries at the same time.
- Lifting weights too quickly
  - This can be harsh on the joints and repetitions should be done in a slow and controlled manner.
- Too little rest or not taking any rest at all.
  - A rest period of one to one and half minutes is recommended between repetitions.
  - Not taking enough rest can cause injury putting a stop to your weight training.

- Not staying hydrated can cause muscles cramp.
  - It is a good idea to carry a bottle of water when you workout
  - Drink lots of water to wash out the impurities from the system
- Working out on an empty stomach.
  - Eat a small and wholesome snack before you workout
  - Leave a gap of at least 30 minutes before you exercise
- Weight-loss does not require weight training
  - Begin your cardio sessions with weight training
  - This will help you start a metabolic burn of calories
  - You can have a gap between the two sessions

Even though instructors may have different opinions about the dos and don'ts of a strength training workout, the most primitive rationale is *playing it safe*. There is no reason for taking unnecessary risks. Once you are aware of the pitfalls and their consequences, avoid making them. Keep your workout simple and at levels you can be in complete control of.

SOME MYTHS ABOUT STRENGTH TRAINING

Strength training comes with its own set of myths, mostly because people are ill-informed about anaerobic exercises.

The goal of strength training is strengthening and building muscle mass. There are many myths that mask this goal. Here we take a look at some of them.

- Women should not lift weights greater than 2 to 3 pounds when exercising
  - This is not true, everyday women lift small children, walk with groceries and run heavy chores around the household.
  - In order to grow bulky muscles, one has to eat lots of food and lift weights. Lifting makes one stronger, not heavier. To gain muscle mass, one has to intake more calories than one expends.
- You can focus on removing fats from specific areas of the body
  - This is not possible. You need to exercise all the muscle groups in order to tone the whole body.
  - When you begin to tone your muscles through strength training, the order of toning cannot be pre-decided as it depends on your body composition.
- Strength training can help you lose weight
  - Not unless you eat right. You have to eat the right amounts of food and remain within the specified calorie limit.

- Lifting weights can be harmful to those with heart disease
  - ◻ If you have read the introduction, you will know that strength training is recommended for a host of illnesses related to the heart, high blood pressure, obesity, high cholesterol and diabetes.
- The same training plan will work for everyone
  - ◻ Since no two people are genetically identical, the same training program may not suit everyone.
  - ◻ Some amount of trial and adjustment is required to find the perfect combination of training and diet that works for you.
  - ◻ Log your effort and calorie intake daily to track your progress and make you accountable.
- Men and women should not do the same strength training
  - ◻ Women can use the same weight machines as men
  - ◻ The goal is to make the muscles lean
- Dieting means starvation
  - ◻ When you do strength training your metabolism rises and you need to eat enough of the right kind of foods
  - ◻ Starving yourself will only make your workout an agony and you will soon lose interest
- Elderly people should not weight train
  - ◻ Strength training is for adults of all ages.
  - ◻ It improves muscle strength and makes flabby muscles lean.
  - ◻ Women at risk for osteoporosis should also weight train; but under the supervision of an expert.

There are numerous myths about strength training. It is always best to do what you enjoy; else you can get sick of it. Remain focused on your workout goals and reward good results to motivate yourself. Making your workout enjoyable ensures that you stick with it.

Don't shy away from trying new things. If you are into strength training using weights and have an interest in running; but have never tried it out, try it for a few weeks as an alternate mode of strength training.

The best things in life are the hardest to get. The best way to fitness is transitioning to an active and healthier lifestyle that you can hold on to for a lifetime.

YOUR HEAD TO TOE STRENGTH WORKOUT

SHOULDERS
- 16 Mack Raises per side/alt
- 16 DB shoulder Press

BICEPS

- 16 DB Curls
- 16 Hammer Curls

TRICEPS

- 16 Tricep Dips
- 16 Tricep Kickbacks per side

CHEST

- 25 Pushups
- 16 DB Bench Presses

BACK

- 16 DB Deadlift w/Single Row
- 16 Single DB Rows per side

ABS

- 12 Rotating T Extensions per side
- 16 Weighted Twists per side/alt

BUTT

- 16 Weighted Bridges
- 16 Donkey Kicks per side

LEGS

- 16 Squat with Side Kick per side
- 16 Standard Squats

CONCLUSION

Today, remaining fit is a major problem. Sedentary lifestyle and eating disorders are some of its causes. As you age, so does your body. Bodily functions deteriorate; there is loss of skeletal muscles mass making you suffer from the lack of physical strength.

A fun test to test your knowledge of strength training

1. It is ok to eat less than 1200 calories when you are strength training.
   a. True
   b. False
2. You need to eat starchy foods when weight training to build muscle mass.
   a. True
   b. False
3. If you are a woman, you cannot lift heavy weights
   a. True
   b. False
4. Strength training will increase your metabolism at rest
   a. True
   b. False
5. If you want to lose weight with strength training, you should eat fewer calories
   a. True
   b. False
6. Building muscle mass with weight training requires that you eat the right calories
   a. True
   b. False

ANSWERS

1. False.
2. True.
3. False.
4. True.
5. False.
6. True.

We have gone into the whys of strength training and explored the best ways possible to accomplish your goal of strengthening your muscles and making them lean.

At this juncture, your knowledge can be put to use in measuring your present fitness and forming an idea about the genre of strength training you would like to do. If you are obese and want to lose weight, strength training will help you achieve your target and keep the gain for long term. If you want to build muscle mass, strength training will help you gain muscle mass. If you want to get stronger and increase your stamina to perform better, strength training will also get you there.

Strength training will help you elevate your metabolism to the levels required for you to perform at peak physical condition. Whether that is at work, at home or in the local sports arena, you will physically improve to do a lot more. Your mental and physical fitness will enable you to live a healthy and active life for a long time.

There is no particular age to begin a fitness regimen, you can start anytime. If you were active and have let your workout slide pressed for time, you can restart now. If you have never worked out before and wondering why you should, it is never too late to start.

The good part of strength training is that you can condition your muscles without having to diet. All that is required is a shift to eating more nutritious and balanced foods. This is the best type of training. It lets you become fit and gradually make a transition to a healthier lifestyle.

If you have read the e-book and are confident that strength training is something you would like to do, then please sign up for a program and get started on your journey to a healthy life!

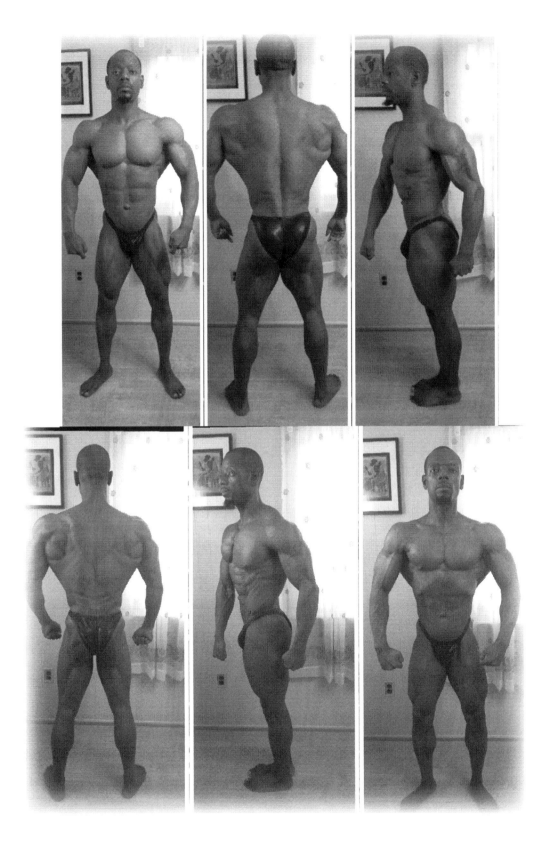

HOW TO GET RIPPED IN JUST 60 DAYS: INTRODUCTION

Most of the men don a desire to have an athletic physique and do a lot to achieve this. However, this is not simple as there are a number of diverse factors that come into play to get a perfect physique. You should follow well established rules to get a well ripped body. Being ripped means to have a body with appropriate balance between body weight and fat. It has been established firmly that your eating habits play a very important role in ripping your body. To achieve the desired look and physique, it is a must to integrate some fat losing exercises.

Body building is the process of strengthening muscles through a variety of exercises and diet programs. This can be achieved by having a well-balanced diet, weight training, muscle conditioning and many other things. Most of the workout sessions are focused on specific muscle categories and the foods that are consumed with the purpose of building the metabolism of your body.

The below chapters will help you know how training and diet can help body builders to achieve their dream goal.

TRAINING

This section focuses on weight, strength and resistance training for body builders. Before you start workout routine, make sure to focus on special exercises that increase the overall mass and have the intention to build the metabolism of your body. To be more specific, people who want to get ripped off should use the technique of contraction where the force of gravity opposes the force generated by the muscles.

Strength training is focused more on increasing the muscular strength that uses weight as a primary force to build the muscle mass. Strength training involves manipulation of sets, reps, tempo and weights that result in a significant increase in size, shape, endurance and strength. Strength training is also known as weight training as it uses weights as key equipment to build mass.

Resistance training involves the use of an elastic resistance, where the muscles are resisting a weight due to which the overall tone of muscles will grow with time. The trainers suggest specific workout for people to begin with, where each workout targets the muscle group.

DIFFERENT TYPES OF TRAINING EXERCISE

Let's have a look at some of the common exercises and training routines that should be followed for overall fitness and body building.

1. Dumb bell bench press

In this kind of exercise, you need to sit on the edge of a flat bench with the dumb-bells resting on the knees. Roll on to the back and bring the dumbbells above the shoulders with palms facing forward. Bend the elbows at 90 degree with the arms parallel to the ground. Press the weights above the center line and keep them under control.

2. Lying triceps push

Sit on a flat bench and hold a curl bar. Lie in such a way that the top of your head is even. Extend the arms over your head and bring the bar directly over your eyes. Keep the elbows tight and upper arms stationary through the training session. Lower the bar slowly till it touches head and press the bar back slowly. Lock the elbow completely to finish the exercise.

3. Preacher curls

This exercise is done on preacher curl bench, where one needs to sit on the edge of the bench and place something firm under their arm pits. Hold the curl bar in the hands with the facing upward and sit as straight as you can. Grasp the bar in hands using a shoulder width grip. Bring the bar up to the chin by putting strain on the muscles to lift the weight.

Lower the bar slowly by putting pressure on the muscles.

4. Dumbbell shrugs

Stand straight with the feet at the width of shoulders. Hold two dumbbells in two hands and droop the shoulders as far as possible. Raise and droop shoulders down as far as possible and return back to the original position. You can even rotate your shoulders in a circular motion holding dumbbells or even barbells.

5. Dumbbell hammer curls

This exercise can be done by holding dumbbells in a standing position with arms hanging at the sides and the palms facing each other. Keep the elbows locked into sides with upper body and elbows in the same place. Curl the weight in right hand with palms facing each other. Avoid turning the wrists during the lift and squeeze the biceps at the top of the lift.

Besides this, you can try a variety of exercises and training routines that include – One-arm dumbbell row, seated dumbbell curl, side lateral dumbbell raise, standing military press, crunches, barbell squat, row, front dumbbell raise, stiff leg barbell, one leg barbell squat, etc. if you have been looking for ways to get a perfect body, *check the online and distant programs* we offer to achieve your dream figure!

DIET AND NUTRITION

The foods you eat play a very impor-tant role in building your muscles. It is a must to pay attention to what you eat, especially if you want to get ripped quickly. Food supplies with calories, which are tiny bits of energy that help the body to perform efficiently. You need a lot of nutrients in the form of vitamins, minerals and carbohydrates to perform your workout.

CARBOHYDRATES

Carbohydrates are an important source of glucose that is stored in the muscles and liver in the form of glycogen. Glycogen can be said as an important form of energy that makes the muscles look and feel full. If you want to get your body ripped in less time, you should include bulk carbohydrates in your diet by focusing more on the unprocessed foods, potatoes, sweet potatoes, oatmeal, whole grain bread, brown rice, etc. The amount of carbs to be taken should be three times your body weight.

GLUCOSE

Glucose provides lot of energy to the brain and helps your body to make blood. Glucose can be made from different sources such as – proteins and carbohydrates. Your body tissues will break down the muscle tissue for glucose, if you are not eating sufficient carbohydrates. It is better to eat more carbs after a workout session such as – refined foods, white rice, sugar, etc that are easy to digest. Intake of high carb after workout session will have less chance of being stored as fat.

PROTEIN

Protein is another important nutrient required by the body builders. Amino acids are the key elements that help the body to build proteins. Protein is very beneficial in growing, repairing and replacing the body tissues and is the basis of the body structure. If the intake of protein exceeds the output, it gets retained in tissues and new muscle mass is added, which is something body builders want. You should concentrate on complete sources of protein such as – fish, eggs, meat, milk etc.

FATS

You need to include fats in your diet, if you want to build a perfect body. Fats are the main source of energy and should be combined with a good source of glucose that spares the breakdown of protein. By including lots of fat-based food items in your diet, you are helping proteins to do their job, which is building muscles. The key to build a perfect body is staying away from bad fat and consuming good fat. It is advised to pay close attention to the fat content of processed food that you eat and try to keep it at minimum. The best type of fat you can include is omega-3 fatty acids and unsaturated fat.

A PERFECT MEAL PLAN

A good diet contains some of the food groups with 5 to 6 smaller meals instead of 3 large meals. You can try out the below mean plan to start with.

1. Vegetable Omelet that is made up of 3 egg whites, 1 cup veggies and 1 whole egg. If you want to increase its protein

value, add some chicken or lean beef.

2. A cup of raw vegetable salad, 1 bagel, 6 oz chicken.

3. 3 packs instant oat meal, 1 cup of yoghurt, 1 banana, 1 cup of cottage cheese

4. 1 piece of fruit and 3-4 oz chicken

5. 1 cup grilled veggies, 1 cup brown rice and 6 oz fish.

6. 2 cups pasta, 8 oz chicken breast, 1 cup yoghurt and 1 apple

When you are trying to build up your body muscles, you need to focus on all kinds of food items. You should be conscious of what you are consuming so that you can maximize your workout sessions.

CONCLUSION

People start body building or ripping their body with the purpose of losing weight. During the workout sessions, they can learn a number of things about what their body is doing and what it is capable of. Overall body building needs a lot of dedication, hard work and commitment towards goals.

It is always better to get started the right way without waiting any longer. Your dream body will be finally the reality!

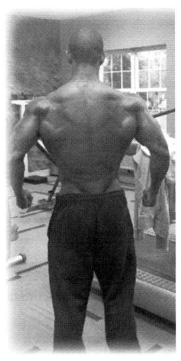
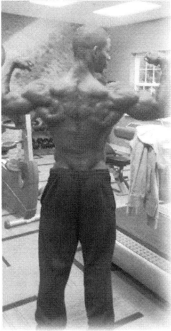

BASICS OF NUTRITION

It actually doesn't matter whether you are aiming to build muscles or to become fitter, there are some basic rules. For example, your diet should be rich in nutrients and you should eliminate as much junk food as possible.

Next up is how much you eat and how much you move your body. If you are in taking a lot of cheese and are stuck to that couch, do not expect to get fit anytime soon. And your diet should be a balanced one, rich in macro as well as micro nutrients.

THE MACRO NUTRIENTS ARE:

Proteins

These are quintessential to muscle building nutrients. In fact, muscles themselves are proteins of some kind. Fish, chicken, liver etc. are rich sources of protein. The vegetarian counterparts consist of pulses, quinoa and soy. You should include at least one thing containing protein with every meal you take in a day. This means you need to include a lot of lean proteins in a diet, which you can get from the above mentioned sources.

Fats

Fats are essential to keep your body moving. Monounsaturated fats are the good fats, which you derive mainly from poultry items. Monounsaturated fats remain liquid at room temperature, for example your oils. Olive oil, peanut oil and canola oils are some examples. Trans-fats, which are there in junk foods in abundance, should be avoided.

Saturated fats are present in the red meat and should be avoided. They are one of the major reasons of obesity and high cholesterol.

Carbohydrates

Carbs are again, good ones as well as bad ones. Simple carbs like sugar are really bad for your body. They cause the sugar level of your blood to plummet and are low in nutrient content. Complex carbs like whole grains are just the opposite. You would have probably heard about something called glycemic index. This is the index, which measures the food intake of carbs that can increase your blood sugar levels. A high glycemic index is considered bad for the body, for obvious reasons.

WHAT IS YOUR BODY TYPE?

Before carving out any strategy for losing your weight, knowing your body type is of utmost importance. Of course, you can't choose your body type; but you can work hard to get a desirable one.

There are 3 types of body:

1. **Ectomorph:**
   These are the people who find it difficult to gain weight. They have stringy muscles, thin limbs and flat chest. Their overall frame is small. They look athletic and have a faster rate of metabolism. They can absorb carbs more easily than the other two body types.

2. **Mesomorph:**
   These people have naturally well-defined muscles. They are athletic too. And they can accumulate muscles easier than the former category. They have a good time being bodybuilders as their body frame is naturally suited to.

3. **Endomorph:**
   These are the people with a broader frame. They are generally heavy on their middle section of the body. They have hard times in losing weight. Thus, your diet should complement your body type.

In fact, your body type can change at different stages of dieting. You need to be aware of these facts before starting up.

Further you should define your nutritional needs. In order to remain energized and lose fat at the same time, you need to have proper ratios of macronutrients in your diet. Just remember that the amount of calories (in kilos) that 1 gram of carb, fat and protein can give you is 4, 9 and 4, respectively.

In order to calculate how much calories you need per day, you should calculate your RMR (Resting Metabolic Rate).

The RMR formula for women is: (10 x weight in kilograms) + (6.25 x height in centimeters[1]) - (5 x age) − 161

Men should use this formula: (10 x weight in kilograms) + (6.25 x height in centimeters) - (5 x age) + 5

Once you have calculated the RMR, multiply this number as per the following rules:

- 1.2 if you have little or no movement at all
- 1.375 if you move a bit
- 1.55 if you exercise moderately
- 1.725 if you are an active exerciser
- 1.9 if you are extremely active in sports and exercise a lot

The general guide for the percentage of total calories as per your body type is:

- Ectomorph: 15 to 20 percent
- Mesomorph: 16 to 21 percent
- Endomorph: 18 to 23 percent

Also, the water intake should be as high as possible. And you must start bunking junk food as much as possible. It is okay to eat 5 times a day in a gap of three to four hours in between. Tea and coffee should be limited. Once a week you can ditch the calorie count and call

---

[1]   1 inch = 2.54 centimeters.

it a cheat day. But it's better to limit the cheat days. And don't starve because if you are keeping yourself hungry, you won't be able to last long in this battle.

You might be thinking of taking in supplements if you are planning to compete. The most effective protein supplements are:

- Whey protein: These are fast actors. Like within 15 minutes of their intake, they will breakdown the amino acids and get absorbed in your blood stream. This has become an all-time favorite protein for all bodybuilders, post workout.
- Casein Protein: Made up of dairy, it is a relatively slower actor. This helps you to keep that feeling of fullness for longer periods of time.
- Egg Protein: It's an excellent source of protein and helps in maintaining the satiety levels for a long period of time.

Final tips on weight loss include a healthy breakfast, which is rich in proteins. It should definitely include one or two fruits. A pre-workout breakfast can have eggs and brown bread. If you are working out on a day, you should definitely include carbs like oatmeal in your breakfast. Baker turkey with boiled vegetables is one healthy breakfast, which the author recommends.

Lunch should be a bit heavy. You should have one more portion of protein in this meal, say chicken steak. Have enough vegetables while lunching.

Dinner should have lean proteins and a lot of veggies. Keep the dinner light.

To avoid sudden pangs of hunger, these three meals should be complimented by snacks at regular intervals. A handful of almonds, a bowl full of blueberries and a fruit salad are good choices of healthy snacks.

THE SELF-CARE CYCLE!

You can burn your body fat by doing aerobic or anaerobic exercises. Aerobic means with air. These exercises leave you gasping for air after 3 minutes. Any exercise, which increases your heart rate, is an aerobic exercise. For instance, jogging, swimming, hopping, skipping etc. You need at least 60 minutes of aerobic exercise to lose some good amount of calories. Anaerobic means without air. Here you need just 30 minutes and that is enough. Remember aerobic is not cardio. Cardio can be both aerobic as well as anaerobic.

THE WORKOUT PLAN

Here the author is sharing her exclusive workout plan for the benefit of the reader:

1. It starts with a warm up exercise, which lasts for 15 minutes at the maximum.
2. Next up is strengthening. Large muscles should be exercised before the smaller ones. You can do pyramids, drop sets, super sets, whatever you like.
3. Cooling down. After you have worked out rigorously, don't head straight for a shower. Just let your muscles relax for a bit.

The final tip the author provides is to properly track your progress. And one should never resort to overtraining. And lastly, set a goal and strive hard to achieve it, with all your will and strength.

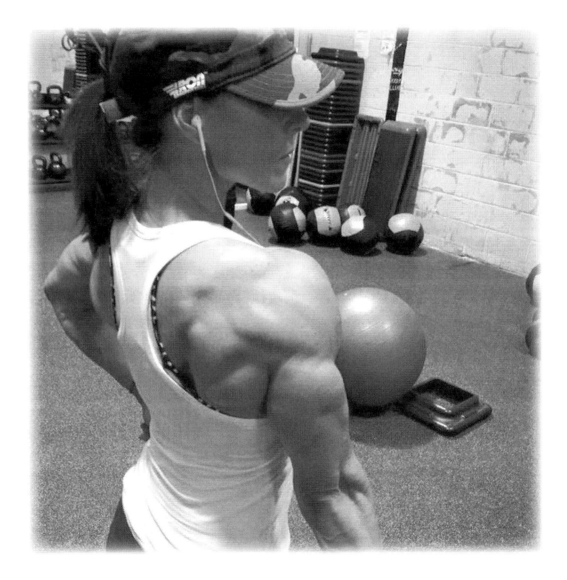

SUPPLEMENTATION: INTRODUCTION

The human body is an amazing development stage in the evolution of the biological life on our earth. The fact that an average mature body has around 37.2 trillion cells is an indicator to its immense complexity. Each part of the body is a combination of different cells. Groups of cells act differently and produce or consume different things to contribute towards the well-being of the entire body. They need different inputs all the time to be able to perform the duties assigned to them. The regular human diet supplies all such inputs to the cells regularly, as and when they are needed, and in the measure they are needed.

The trillions of body cells require thousands of different things every moment. Diets of communities all over the world have evolved over the ages to contain everything the body cells need. Anybody having such a balanced diet regularly is unlikely to need any special dietary supplement. But sometimes, the diet may not provide everything the body needs in the right quantity. Some regions and diets may be deficient in a specific nutrient. Hunger and poverty may deprive a significant chunk of the population of a balanced diet as also the sufficient amount of nutrition. Some persons may be averse to eating something that provides some vital nutrients to their body. If they refuse to eat that essential thing for long, they will eventually develop a deficiency of that particular nutrient in the body. This can prove to be harmful for the body.

Such an eventuality creates the need of dietary supplements. These include vitamins, minerals, fiber, fatty acids and amino acids. These are usually consumed in the form of a pill, capsule, tablet or liquid. These are no food substitutes nor are they intended to treat a particular disease. In general, dietary supplements are to be avoided. When one becomes necessary, it must be taken only after consultation with the doctor.

Thousands of dietary supplements are produced and marketed aggressively across the world. The commercial world is run on profit. It presents facts about dietary supplements in such a manner that innumerable persons begin to feel that these are absolutely essential for the well-being of the body. The advertisements keep speaking about the needs of growing children, pregnant women, lactating mothers, aging persons, body-builders and muscle-builders in normal as well as unusual working conditions like during times of strain and tension. Many people are tempted to use these supplements after seeing such campaigns, without consulting their doctors. So do go in for a diet supplement only when it becomes necessary. The right use of supplements in the appropriate situations will make sure you can stay healthier and longer without any health issues.

DIFFERENT NUTRIENTS THAT YOU CAN GET FROM SUPPLEMENTS

The human body needs different nutrients to survive and to function. It cannot synthesize essential nutrients like carbohydrates, fat, proteins, vitamins and minerals. The diet has to supply these nutrients to the body regularly and in sufficient quantities. Foods provide the calories, which fuel the body. Water is instrumental in maintaining the internal conditions in the body. It carries nutrients to the cells and plays a part in the disposal of the body's waste products. The brain gets its energy mainly from carbohydrates. Water and carbohydrates are provided in the diet.

All other nutrients can be provided by dietary supplements. These include minerals, amino acids, vitamins, organ tissues, enzymes, metabolites and concentrates. These are usually marketed in the form of capsules, tablets, liquids, powders, bars, sprays or gels.

AMINO ACIDS

These are made of amine (-NH2) and carboxylic acid (-COOH) groups. They also have a side-chain, distinct for each amino acid. Amino acids go into the making of all proteins and nearly 20 percent of the body is formed by them. They also play a part in the transportation and storage of nutrients. They are needed during the healing of wounds and repair of tissues. There are three types of amino acids: essential, non-essential and conditional. The body cannot make the essential amino acids and has to get them from food. The body makes non-essential amino acids by using essential amino acids or from proteins. Conditional amino acids are required during sickness like cancer.

VITAMINS

Body needs small quantities of vitamins from external sources as it cannot synthesize them. The body needs 2 types of vitamins: fat-soluble vitamins and water-soluble vitamins. Blood carries water-soluble vitamins to all the cells, where they are absorbed, whenever necessary. When they are not needed, they are excreted through urine. Body fat stores fat-soluble vitamins for up to 6 months. The water soluble vitamins include B1 (thiamin), B12, folate, B6, B2 (riboflavin), niacin, biotin, pantothenic acid and vitamin C. The fat-soluble vitamins are A, D, E and K.

PROTEINS

Proteins play a vital role in the growth and maintenance of the body tissues.

They are needed to produce hormones and enzymes, which control most body functions. When necessary, protein can also supply energy to the body. Lean protein should provide 10 to 35 percent of the daily calorie needs of the body.

MINERALS

The body requires substances like calcium, chloride, fluoride, iron, magnesium, phosphorus, potassium, sodium and zinc in various proportions. Sodium and potassium are needed for the regulation of fluid processes in and around the cell. Calcium is required to build and maintain the bones and teeth. Iron is needed for building muscles and maintaining the health of blood. The body also needs elements like copper, chromium, iodine, manganese, molybdenum and selenium in traces.

ESSENTIAL FATTY ACIDS

The body needs essential fatty acids to maintain good health; but cannot synthesize them. Fatty acids can yield large quantities of ATP and are preferred as fuel by the heart and skeletal muscle cells.

BODYBUILDING SUPPLEMENTS

Athletes and body builders use bodybuilding supplements, sometimes to replace their meals. These are aimed at gaining or losing weight, building muscle mass and strength and for improving their performance.

The more popular dietary supplements are vitamins, protein drinks, amino acids, glutamine, essential fatty acids, creatine and weight gain or loss products.

WHY ARE THESE NUTRIENTS NECESSARY FOR OUR HEALTH?

A deficiency of nutrients occurs when the body does not get the required amount of vitamins and minerals. Nutritional deficiencies adversely affect the cellular functions and processes like water balance, nerve signaling, digestion, enzyme activity and metabolism. They can lead to diseases like osteoporosis or anemia, caused respectively by the deficiency of calcium and iron. They can also lead to health issues like indigestion, defective bone growth, skin problems and dementia.

Nutritional deficiencies may show up through general symptoms like weakness, sleepiness, breathing trouble, constipation, fatigue, depression and poor concentration. Such indications are often ignored. But these indicate a serious nutritional deficiency. If you are not having a regular balanced diet, are not eating regularly or are eating overcooked food, the role of supplements becomes more vital. Your body can get the required amount of nutrients through these supplements.

Stress is a common phenomenon in everybody's life today. It is dangerous for the body. It affects the body's immune system. Supplements provide the nutritional backup that keeps the body defenses at the optimum level. Various deficiencies lead to a different malfunctioning of the body. Supplements are necessary to prevent such deficiencies and keep the body working at the best possible levels.

Vitamin deficiencies can cause many health problems. The health of our bones depends upon Vitamin D. Its deficiency shows up through muscle pain and fatigue. Bone softening is the outcome of a prolonged deficiency. The use of vitamin D supplement can ease this situation. Vitamin B12 has a role in the production of the brain's neurotrans-mitters and DNA. Its deficiency causes numbness in the legs, hands, or feet. There can be some difficulty in walking and balance. Anemia and fatigue are also common. Vitamin B12 supplements can relieve these symptoms. A folate deficiency leads to a reduced number of cells and neural tube defects in a fetus. Its symptoms are mouth ulcers, fatigue and gray hair. So, pregnant women need folic acid supplements that are to be taken on a daily basis.

Calcium's role in the development and functions of the bones, muscles and the nerves is vital. Very low calcium causes fatigue, muscle cramps and loss of appetite. A regular calcium supplement keeps such problems away. Potassium has a big part to play in the proper func-tioning of the heart, kidneys and other organs. Diarrhea or vomiting and profuse sweating can cause short-term potassium deficiency. This causes muscle weak-ness, weight loss and constipation. To overcome these problems, potassium supplements are necessary.

Iron is required in the making of the red blood cells. Low iron levels means that the body cannot carry enough oxygen. Supplements are necessary to boost the iron levels. Magnesium is needed for good bone health. It has a role in energy production as well. Its deficiency can cause nausea, vomiting and loss of appetite. This can end up in muscle cramps and seizures. Supplements help to restore health.

Thus, the deficiency of every nutrient leads to some health problem in the body. Diet supplements help the body to overcome such problems and allow it to stay fit.

FOODS THAT CONTAIN NUTRIENTS

The human body needs vitamins, minerals, fiber, fatty acids and amino acids every day, in addition to water and carbohydrates. Fresh fruits, milk products, vegetables, whole grains, nuts and seeds, legumes, fishes and lean meats are health foods, rich in vitamins, minerals, essential fatty acids and fiber. Most of them are whole foods. They do not need much processing, nor have any artificial ingredients. They are readily available everywhere and are priced reasonably. And the best thing about them is they not only taste great; but also have an attractive flavor.

FRUITS AND VEGETABLES

Low in fat, fruits and vegetables bring lot of nutrients and variety to the diet. Colorful, dark green and orange fruits and vegetables have more nutrients.

Blueberries are full of antioxi-dants, including anthocyanins and phytochemicals. They lower blood pressure in over-weight adults with metabolic syndrome. They reduce oxidized LDL cholesterol and aid in the fight against cancer. Pineapple offers vitamin C, minerals, vitamin B, some enzymes and fiber. They lower blood pressure, fight cancer and contribute towards keeping the bowel habits regular. Strawberries contain substantial vitamin C, which keeps teeth and gums in excellent conditions. They have fiber that promotes digestion and their flavonoids fight cancers.

Green vegetables like spinach and fenugreek have vitamin K, protein, fiber, pro-vitamin A - carotenoid, vitamin C, folate and manganese. Garlic is full of vitamins C, B1 and B6, allicin, calcium, copper, potassium, selenium and manganese. It reduces blood pressure and LDL cholesterol. Garlic kills bacteria and fungi.

Potatoes have potassium, iron, copper, magnesium and manganese in good measure along with vitamin C and B. They contain almost every nutrient the body needs in small measures. Sweet potatoes have a good amount of potassium and vitamin A.

Peanuts are full of protein and mono and polyunsaturated fats. They lower the risk of cardiovascular disease and type 2 diabetes.

DAIRY PRODUCTS

Milk products have 16 nutrients including calcium, vitamin D and proteins. Milk, cheese and yogurt also have potassium and probiotics. Milk products also contribute phosphorus, vitamins A and B12, riboflavin and niacin.

Grains

Low in fat, whole-grain foods have fiber, carbohydrates, protein, vitamins and minerals. Nutrient-rich beans have proteins, fiber and phytonutrients. They protect the body from diabetes, cardiovascular diseases and cancers. They build and repair the muscles. Sunflower seeds contain monounsaturated and polyunsaturated fats, protein, fiber, vitamin E, folate, thiamin, niacin and iron.

POULTRY AND FISH

The fat content of chicken is low and its protein content is high. It can be eaten in many healthy ways like baking and roasting. The egg yolk has vitamins, minerals and other nutrients. They have antioxidants like lutein and zeaxanthine, which protect the eyes and lower the risk of eye diseases. It also has choline and healthy fats. Fishes have protein, omega-3 fatty acids, vitamins D and B2, calcium, iron, zinc, phosphorus, potassium, iodine and magnesium.

MEAT

Choose low-fat, lean cuts of beef or pork. Trim outside fat before cooking. Trim any inside, separable fat before eating. Baking, broiling and roasting are the healthiest ways to prepare meat. It is best to limit how often you eat beef, pork, veal and lamb, because even lean cuts contain a lot of fat and cholesterol when compared to other protein sources. Meats of various types have proteins, fat, vitamins and minerals in varying degrees. Liver has the most vitamins, proteins, copper, phosphorus, zinc, iron and selenium.

MUSHROOMS

Mushrooms have plenty of selenium, which fights cancer. They also have vitamin D, copper and potassium.

Including these food items in our daily diet will ensure that the body gets all the essential nutrients in balanced amounts and keep us healthy and fit.

THINGS TO AVOID TO ENSURE OPTIMUM NUTRITION OF THE BODY

It is possible that some people may not be regularly eating a wide variety of nutritious foods. They may be better off if they take some supplements, which provide a sufficient quantum of the missing nutrients. Some supplements are good for general health: for example; Calcium and vitamin D keep the bones strong and cut down on the bone loss, folic acid reduces the risk of birth defects and omega-3 fatty acids ease the heart conditions. But, it is obvious that supplements cannot replace a healthy and balanced diet. So the first and the most vital thing nobody should do is to ignore eating a balanced and nutritious diet on a regular basis.

THE FOLLOWING ARE SOME OF THE DON'TS FOR THE PEOPLE WHO USE DIETARY SUPPLEMENTS.

- Do not take new supplements without being ready for the side effects because the active ingredients in supplements can have strong effects in the body.
- Do not replace prescribed medicines with supplements. Do not use multiple supplements together without medical advice: Vitamin K affects the effectiveness of blood thinner coumadin in preventing blood clotting. Antioxidants like vitamins C and E impact the effectiveness of chemotherapy. Many such unexpected complications can occur with the intake of multiple supplements.
- Do not take supplements without ensuring that they do not lead to excess intake of some nutrients, which may also be available in your daily diet. Many supplements are being added to various cereals and beverages. Note that more of nutrients will not always be better. Apart from expenses, they can lead to side effects.
- Pregnant or nursing mothers must not go beyond the multivitamin and mineral supplements unless prescribed by a doctor. Do not take supplements after diagnosing your health condition yourself. Do not take an overdose of any supplement.

HERE ARE SOME OF THE DOS

Some supplements are necessary in special situations. Pregnant women need extra folic acid, vitamins and iron. Fifty plus adults need more of vitamin B-12 through fortified cereals or a multivitamin supplement. Persons aged 65 and more need extra vitamin D daily to cut down the risk of injuries through falls.

People eating significantly less than the average intake may need some supplements. Vegetarians, whose diet may not have sufficient variety of foods, may have to opt for some supplements. Women experiencing heavy bleeding during the menstrual period will need some supplements. People with a chronic condition which affects their capacity to absorb or use nutrients may need vitamin supplements regularly.

Whatever the supplements you make take, it is advisable to maintain a record of their effects and convey them to your doctor periodically. After all, the purpose of supplements is to reduce the problems faced by the body, not to increase them. It is best to consult an expert who can prescribe you the most potent supplement based on your specific condition.

SOME MYTHS ASSOCIATED WITH NUTRITION

Millions of people keep taking some supplement or the other for a long period in their life. Although some supplements are genuinely necessary, they may not be required at all in some cases. All that could be necessary is to easily modify the diet of the person. But dietary supplements have become a big business across the world. The motive of the commercial world is continuous growth in production and the sales of goods for increasing profits. Aggressive advertisement campaigns are always singing praises of new and newer versions of more potent and magical dietary supplements. The dietary supplement industry has always believed in creating enduring myths about the dire need of super-acting supplements. Such myths are often reinforced by relatives, friends and neighbors, who talk of the astonishing results of various supplements.

- One of the popular claims by every producer of a supplement is that scientists, professionals and doctors have found it extremely effective or that a survey has shown excellent results. But none of these claims is substantiated by evidence. There is no mention of these scientists or experts and the credibility of the surveys is always doubtful. Every such claim has to be judged on the basis of hard evidence, for or against it.

- The marketing wings of supplements love to spread the idea that various studies have shown that their supplements have been producing fantastic results. The attempt is to create an impression that clinical research has proved the effectiveness of their product. However, the methods

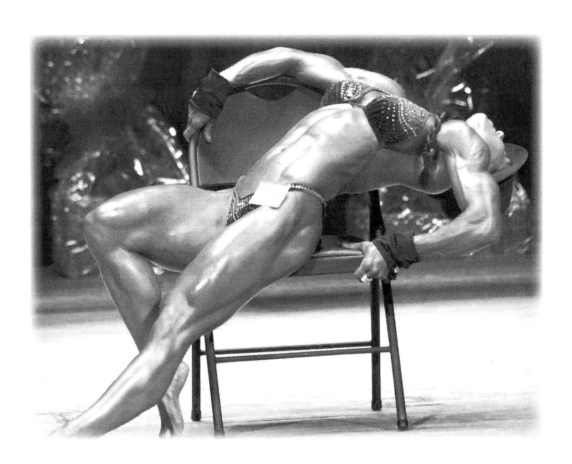

adopted are often ill-defined and there is no control group for observing the effects of the supplement. The results and the claims based on such methods can never be reliable.

- There is an impression among a section of people that supplements can prevent diabetes or heart disease. This is obviously an erroneous impression. No supplement is meant to treat a specific disease. It is merely a nutritional additional to the diet. It cannot achieve anything more.

- Another general misconception is that the best supplements are natural products. Consumers are attracted by labels which claim that all the ingredients of this product are natural. The marketing wizards keep harping on the idea that the natural products in their supplement are safe and there cannot be anything better than these natural products. This is all misleading. The basic need of the supplement is felt because of the deficiency of a nutrient. If that deficiency is overcome, it does not matter whether the product is natural or not. What matters is its nutritional efficacy.

- Yet another flawed argument is that something is being

used for ages and so, it must be good. There was no way to assess the effects of a treatment over a long period until the beginning of the modern era. What has been used all these years may or may not pass the test today. Every supplement has to be tested extensively to determine its effects over the short and long terms. Only then, it can be cleared for general use.

- Many people believe that the multivitamins and calcium supplements are the same. But it should be noted that each supplement acts differently. They may not even be similar. The belief that all the supplements for sale are approved for sale is also not true. Authorities begin investigation only when some complaints are lodged against a product. Some people tend to think that supplements can take care of a poor diet. They are wrong. Supplements are not an alternative to a good diet.

Hence, it is extremely important that people use the supplements that have a well proved backing from reliable sources and have been authenticated by a competent body for their effectiveness in managing a deficiency.

CONCLUSION

A regular intake of essential nutrients in the right amount is necessary for maintaining the human body in good health. So the identification and isolation of nutrients in pure form had fueled the hopes that vitamin and mineral supplements will take care of our general health. Nutrient supplements are as important as the balanced diet in maintaining health.

Even earlier, the experts were divided over the use of supplement versus a balanced diet debate. Many have been arguing that the most important thing is to have a wholesome, varied and balanced diet full of nutrients. The supplements should come into picture only when the balanced diet fails to provide all the nutrients in adequate quantities.

However, it is obvious that some persons do derive benefit from supplements. It is clear that vitamin D and calcium supplements do prevent the onset of osteoporosis. Omega-3 fatty acids do reduce the risk of cardiovascular diseases. And fluoride prevents teeth cavities in children.

Hence, people are advised to use the supplements judiciously and also make sure that they eat a well-balanced diet so that each and every organ in their body functions at an optimum level.

METABOLISM: INTRODUCTION

Exercising your body grows in importance as you age. Getting older has manifold effect on our bodies and one of them is how it affects the metabolism.

Metabolism is a very important process in the human body. It is a set of chemical reactions that are required to release the energy contained in the food we eat so that our bodies can use it to fuel its activities. These activities include everything that our body requires to remain functional, for example walking, digesting food and growing.

If you are obese and searching for ways to shed the fat, then ways to boost metabolism in order to release large amounts of energy from your body by burning the fat is necessary. Or, if you are an elderly person, then finding ways to increase metabolism is beneficial for your good health and for maintaining the required level of activity.

In the aging process, we lose muscle mass. Our daily activities make us use our skeletal muscles and keep them oxygenated. However, if you wish to maintain your body and remain lean and fit over the years, you need to work on your muscles. Building muscle mass is an excellent way for the body to improve its metabolism.

Physical activity that goes beyond daily chores and work schedule and takes you to a park, inside a gym or on the bike path is a habit that has to be cultivated, if you wish to transition to a lifestyle that includes regular exercise.

An active lifestyle with regular aerobic and anaerobic exercises is recommended to control and prevent many chronic diseases like diabetes and osteoporosis.

Educating yourself about exercising to boost your metabolism is necessary if you are planning to lose weight. Anaerobic exercises build muscle mass. Anaerobic means *without air*. For example, lifting heavy weights in the gym would leave you gasping for air within a few minutes. The muscles are strained and require more energy to lift the weight. The body is forced to create a metabolic spike to release the energy. The heart has to pump faster to meet the additional demand for the oxygenated blood to the muscles thereby increasing the heart rate. The increased demand on the heart makes the heart muscles strong and resilient to heart diseases. Having a strong heart is beneficial for long term health.

Metabolic exercises are a more holistic approach to a workout than just aerobic exercises. A judicious mix of aerobic and anaerobic exercises is required to maintain the weight-loss gained last for a long time.

For those who lead a sedentary lifestyle, inculcating a habit of performing metabolic exercises for at least 20 to 40 minutes, 2 or 3 times a week, will be beneficial. The metabolism will remain elevated for a long time after the session is over and continue to release calories from the body.

It should be noted that any exercise regimen should be started only after consulting a doctor and having a thorough check up.

THE BEST WAYS TO IMPROVE YOUR METABOLISM – THROUGH EXERCISE

Whether you are an exercise-lover and workout daily or are planning on starting on a weight-loss regimen, there are a few things you need to know about the effect of exercise on your metabolism. What you may not know is that different exercises affect your metabolic rate differently. If you are planning on doing exercises regularly, it will impact your metabolic rate.

Aerobic exercise being the easiest regimen attracts the most people. You can walk, run or go to a gym to use cardio machines and workout. This form of exercise will help you lose body weight, but will not help sustain this weight loss by keeping your metabolism elevated afterwards.

Anaerobic training which is far more intensive done in 20 to 40 minute sessions *will* keep your metabolism spike up even after the session is over. As muscles are able to burn more fat calories, it is a good way to develop a lean body with strong muscles. Metabolic exercises can help you raise your energy levels, make your skeletal muscles lean as well as induce weight loss. When accompanied by a proper diet, the effect of metabolic exercise can become manifold.

Metabolic exercises can be done with or without any equipment, using just a pair of dumbbells. You can decide with your fitness instructor on a set of special exercises that are aimed to make the muscles do the work. Then repeat these exercises in sets of 5 or more as instructed. An exercise may be a single move or a combination of moves.

The following is a list of exercises and the area of the body they affect:

- Exercise while swinging a weight - like a dumbbell – held in each hand, moving gently forward and backward in tandem with the given exercise or as directed
  - Leg kicks forward and back will work to tone the triceps, butt and thighs
  - Squats with the weights held at an angle will act to tone the muscles of the shoulder and upper back muscles along with arms, butt and thighs

- ❑ Knee bends. Lying face up with knees bent, raising the abs and joining the hands above the chest to tone the abs and chest muscles
- ❑ Push press to tone the muscles of the arms, legs and the abs

- The above are example of exercises used for creating sophisticated set of moves that have been tested and recommended by experienced metabolic exercise trainers and are effective when accompanied by the recommended diet. However, being technical exercises, they are very exhausting and can have you out of breadth and tire your body long before you can expect any sort of metabolic response.

- High Intensity Cardio
  - ❑ This type of cardio exercise will create metabolic spikes and continue to burn fat after the session has ended. This is good for weight loss as well as for maintaining the weight-loss gained in the long term. These exercises being very tough on the body should be interspersed with few rest days. Cardio exercises affect all parts of the body.

- Weight Training
  - ❑ Weight training is the cornerstone of metabolic exercise and can be done at different levels. The best weight training equipment always comes with many levels of control. This allows you to adjust weights to levels you are comfortable with.

  - ❑ When cardio-vascular exercise is followed by this type of metabolic training that builds and strengthens the muscles, it maximizes your weight loss efforts. This is recommended for long term to permanent weight loss maintenance.

  - ❑ Supervised, high intensity weight training can burn up to ten fat calories per minute with rest periods of thirty seconds to one minute in between. These training sessions need to have adequate rest periods of at least one day in between.

  - ❑ Weight training equipment is made specifically for different muscle groups of the body. There are machines for tightening the muscles of the abdomen, others stretch the spinal cord and work on the upper body. Yet others can be used to train the upper arm, shoulders and the leg muscles.

  - ❑ It is a good idea to have a workout routine that makes you give some time to a variety of machines such that all the different muscle groups are exercised in turn.

- Running and sprinting interval training
  - Professional runners use this kind of interval training to strengthen the leg muscles. You should consult an experienced trainer for advice on this method of metabolic training and find out what level of endurance is suitable for you.

The above high-intensity cardio workouts will boost your metabolism for periods of at least 24 hours after the session. The muscle mass gained during the program will be lean and make your body strong helping you perform better. The advantage is that the weight loss will be maintained for a long time.

FOODS THAT CAN BOOST YOUR METABOLISM

A metabolic diet allows you to vary your diet so that the goal of eating fewer calories to lose the fat may be reached quickly.

Metabolism is the rate of cellular oxidation or simply said; the speed at which food gets converted to energy. Metabolism varies from person to person. In some people, metabolism takes place faster than in others.

People who are fast oxidizers need to eat more proteins to slow down their metabolism, while those who are slow oxidizers need to eat more carbohydrates

to crank up their metabolism. What is your metabolic type can only be answered by a physician using your urine and blood sample test results.

According to researcher William Wolcott in his book "The Metabolic Typing Diet" says that people can be categorized into three common metabolic types: the protein-types, the carbo-types and the mixed-types. However, as metabolic diets are prescribed for disease prevention by doctors, anyone seeking to use these diets for weight-loss should first get an approval from a physician.

The foods that can be found in different types of metabolic diets are as follows

PROTEIN TYPES

- Diets whose major components are protein fats and oils
- Many call this a weight loss Atkins diet that is rich in proteins

CARBO TYPES

- Rich in carbohydrates with little protein and fats

MIXED TYPES

- This diet is a mix of high protein, fats and carbohydrates

A metabolic diet is very specific to the individuals' metabolic needs and is not the same for everyone. It depends upon the body composition, which is the proportion of fat and fat-free mass. Fat-free mass is made up of lean muscle, our organs, tissue and water all of which are given and cannot be varied.

Walcott further says that a metabolic diet, if not correctly prescribed, can disturb the body's oxidation process and adversely affect the metabolic rates by lowering it. *Click here to buy the supplements* that will help you get the best nutrition so that you can achieve better health and fitness.

Even though a metabolic diet has become a very popular compliment to anaerobic cardio for weight-loss, critics of metabolic diet have cautioned about the fundamental structure of this *diet* as not being balanced.

Recent studies have shown that dieters who take more protein than carbs tend to lose weight, gain muscle mass and are more lean and fit. Given this the question is how much protein should you take?

In a study of obese women, a 30% protein diet and high dairy diet as opposed to those whose diet contained comparatively less protein and dairy, it was seen that the high protein group lost more weight and grew lean muscles. The high protein diet kept the metabolism elevated even when inactive or at rest.

The author of the above study then suggests that in order to build lean muscles that would help keep the weight-loss gained in the long run; a protein rich diet is necessary. Lean muscles burn calories even when the body is at rest.

Considering that ultimately calories have to be burned for weight-loss, whether they are from protein or fat is not important. A transition to healthy eating is necessary along with an interest to educate yourself about foods that will seamlessly help you lose weight and make you feel good at the same time when you add them to your daily diet, for example green tea and dairy.

If you are planning on selecting a metabolic diet for weight-loss, make sure that you consult your physician before you begin.

WHAT YOU SHOULD NOT DO WHILE PERFORMING METABOLISM-BOOSTING EXERCISES

Metabolic exercises can become very intensive and one should be careful to avoid injuries. Added to this are metabolic diets whose long term effects are relatively unknown. So with the help of some research here is a summarized list of what you should not do.

- Jumping exercises can cause injuries
  - If you are doing intense exercises that involve jumping up and down from a height like a box, using both legs, please remember that it can be very hard on the joints. To avoid knee injury, jump down using one leg at a time.
- Exercising using the *no pain no gain* as a rule of the thumb should be avoided

- Don't work so intensely that your body becomes sore and that you can hardly walk. You are unable to move and have to rest a few days for the soreness to go away. Fitness experts advise that you work out within your physical limits.
- Also, intense exercising requires that you take a day of rest in between.
- Adding weight training to your exercise regimen will help you stretch, build and strengthen the muscles *gently*, which is a good way to improve your metabolism

- Technical exercises could make your efforts to raise your metabolism tedious
  - These exercises require a great deal of flexibility and practice before they can be repeated enough times to be effective as metabolic exercises
  - It is easier to do aerobic dancing or brisk walking. Both are as effective and do not require the sort of agility required for technical exercises

- American Heart Association does not support high protein diet for weight loss
  - AHA does not support diets that are high in protein and low on carbohydrates as a means to losing weight

- Such diets are not balanced and can cause serious *"metabolism dysfunction"* in people without them being even aware of it
- The origins of metabolic diets lie in their use for disease control. Using them for weight loss could lead to other problems

- Continue a metabolic diet for as long as you want is a big no
  - This is true. A metabolic diet continued over a long period of time is not recommended.
  - Advocates of the diet recommend a maximum of one month and consider it more of a transition to a new lifestyle
  - It has been seen that in most cases people on metabolic diets tend to resume their previous eating habits.

- Beginning a metabolic diet regimen without consulting a physician, is not recommended
  - If you have read this far you should be aware of the pros and cons of this diet.
  - A protein rich metabolic diet could create serious problems for diabetics
  - It is absolutely necessary to consult a physician before starting a metabolic diet

- If you are obese and want to lose weight quickly, then consider transitioning to a fitter lifestyle with regular exercise and a diet that is balanced and nutritious. Building muscles using resistance training is the best way to sustain any gain in weight-loss over a long period of time.

SOME MYTHS ABOUT METABOLISM AND METABOLIC RATE

Metabolism is often misinterpreted by dieters eager to shed pounds as quickly as possible as the main culprit in weight gain. However this is not entirely true. We use energy all the time, even as we sleep the heart beats and the lungs breathe. Metabolism is the process which works continuously to produce energy required by the body.

Further, the body composition affects the metabolism rates more than anything else. Some people are just *fastburners* of food while other are *slow burners*. Also, having many small meals will not affect the rate of metabolism.

According to a well-researched article written by *physical instructor Jeremy Duvall*, the following are some of the best known myths about metabolism.

- Thinner people have higher metabolism
  - Often, we find thin people are able to eat as much as they want without having to worry about the *carbs*. This is not because they have a

high metabolism, but most likely because their body composition has lower fat mass.

- When at rest, their metabolism *slows* down as there is very little fat to burn.
- On the flip side, people who are overweight have higher metabolism when they are at rest as they have large fat mass.
- Further, comparing two people having equal weights where one of them has leaner muscles, the latter would have a higher rate of metabolism as lean muscles tend to burn fat faster.
- Thus, we can safely say that it is the *body composition* that affects the rate of metabolism more than any other factor like size

- Eating many small meals will improve your metabolism
  - This is not true. Eating small meals every 4 hours is a way for dieters to control their cravings. Frequent eating does not translate to higher metabolism.
  - However, the sum total of calories you take has to be within the specified limit and whether it is taken in one sitting or over several small meals does not make much of a difference.

- What is more important is the kind of food that you consume and how much of it. If you are prone to eating fried foods and desserts. then your fat mass will increase and not your muscles; if you are a weight watcher, this will affect your weight loss goals.
- Inculcating good eating habits will be more useful in the long run and is therefore a better goal than trying to control metabolism.

- There are no ways for you to control your metabolism
  - This is not entirely true, studies have shown that you can have some control over your metabolism
  - You can do this by building muscles and making your fatty muscles lean
  - Sleep induces fat metabolism and it is recommended that one sleeps for at least 7½ hours every day. Sleep also reduces stress and hunger and increases vitality
  - Drinking water is another way to burn fat as opposed to sweetened drinks that add calories.
  - Coffee adds caffeine to the body providing an energy boost any time of the day.
  - Finally, a protein and dairy-rich diet has been proven to make a difference in the metabolism, enough to lose weight.
  - Simple pleasures in life like a cup of green tea burn calories significantly at rest.

Making smart adjustments to your diet along with exercising with weights to force your muscles to work and grow can stimulate the metabolism that will work even at rest.

CONCLUSION

According to studies done on metabolic exercise, they can be done in three different intensities: light, moderate and heavy. The higher the intensity; the greater will be the calories released, the greater will be the weight loss.

Activities that are a combination of aerobic exercise and require overcoming resistance like aerobic dancing, snow shoveling and biking at speeds of 20 to 30 kilometers per hour can turn into high intensity anaerobic exercises.

Advocates of metabolic diet promise lasting changes in lifestyle and diet. The AHA along with a host of other health conscious organizations does not support a protein rich, low carbohydrate diet. These diets being controversial in nature should be considered after checking with a doctor first.

Answer the following questions to test your understanding of metabolism.

1. Technical exercise is easier than brisk walking
   a. True

b. False
2. Weight training does not help build muscles mass
   a. True
   b. False
3. Muscles induce metabolism to continue burning fat even at rest
   a. True
   b. False
4. It has been seen that metabolic diets can be used to burn fat
   a. True
   b. False
5. Metabolic diets can be continued for a long period of time
   a. True
   b. False
6. One can maximize weight-loss effort with a combination of metabolic diet and exercise
   a. True
   b. False

ANSWERS

1. False. Technical exercise requires agility and practice to master them. The effort can exhaust you physically way before you begin to burn any calories.
2. False. Resistance provided to the muscles through weight training help to build muscles.
3. True. Lean muscles elevate metabolism to burn fat and release energy even at rest.
4. True. However being controversial in nature, it is best to get a physician's approval first.
5. False. These diets are not balanced and should be used for very short periods of time
6. Both true and false. Metabolic exercise done along with weight training works to make the weight loss gains last for a long time. Metabolic diets should be used with caution. It is less stressful to go on a regular diet that inculcates good eating habits.

Having read this far, you will have formed a good idea about metabolism and things you should consider before starting a metabolic program. When you make your program choices, it is a good idea to remember to assess your strengths and choose those workouts that you can adjust to easily without losing your rhythm, confidence and balance. If you have never worked out before, loosen up with stretches to flex your muscles, use a treadmill or just walk fast to build your leg muscles and pull some weights for stamina.

At the same time, try making small changes to your diet that will be beneficial to you in the long run. Eating foods with less fat will improve your cholesterol levels and protect you from saturated fats. Another pitfall to avoid is sugary foods and desserts. These and many more small changes like substituting polished grains with whole grains will make your diet leaner and more metabolic naturally.

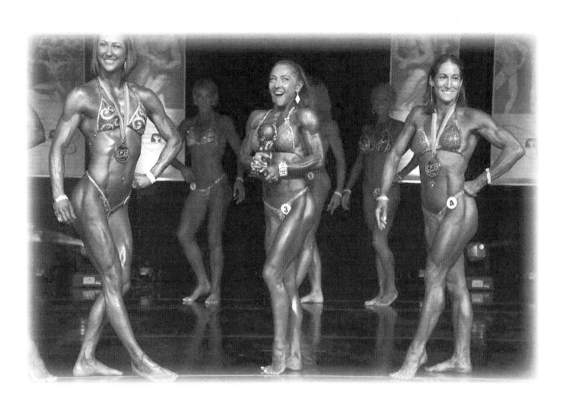

METABOLISM REHAB

In case you are not aware of the harsh reality, it should be pointed out that unskilled and inexperienced coaches may put you in situations where you not only end up losing money; but also injure yourself. Rather it is more important that one invests in courses where results are given more importance than the use of advanced equipment and not just the gimmicks and flashes. One common complaint, which is generally received from clients, is that the training methodology for everyday clients and athletes remains the same and they consider it as "one program for all". They should also consider the long term risks involved here which can lead to many injuries and later can be dangerous as well may very well deter an average person to continue the same without any workout program.

This book has been written keeping many a things in mind and the most important of them is keeping the requirement of the client and his results at the top of the list. It was drafted with the sole intention that even an average person would be able to make it out supported by proven techniques as well as advises that would surely benefit all.

NOW COMING TO AN IMPORTANT PART OF THIS BOOK: THE METABOLISM

One of the biggest mistakes people normally make while cutting for a competitions is that they take naive advice and end up consuming less calories presumable as a part of their newly crafted diet plan. This overall process pulls down metabolism which is nothing but the chemical processes that are continuously going on inside the body to keep us alive and active. The minimum energy which the body would require to carry out the mentioned chemical processes is known as Basal Metabolic Rate and it ranges between 40% – 70% of the body's energy requirement. Basal Metabolic Rate is always low for people with high fat content and more muscle content. Likewise overweight people will always have high BMR than their lean counterparts as the same would be required to maintain a large body size.

Referring to the need of increasing BMR for our day to day activities, it may also be pointed out that it is important to increase the BMR to lose weight. But the mere presence of artificial products actually makes it extremely difficult to distinguish between fiction and facts. However, as a solution to this problem, we have given exhaustive details on our website *www.teamhardbodycoaching.com* about ways and means for increasing BMR. The three most active ways to increase BMR are aerobic activities, strength training and high intensity interval training.

Aerobic exercises are considered to be the most effective ways of burning calories. Most common types include swimming, cycling and walking. Ideal amount of time which is considered for this is 150 minutes per week along with the necessary changes in the diet. Under strength training, focus is always on burning muscle tissues than fat tissues and involves high intensity body exercises and lifting weights. Last but not the least, HIIT or high intensity interval training is all about increasing the metabolic rate even after the exercise is over.

There are many ways of keeping the body active by having an ideal BMR rate. Some of those are mentioned below:

Building muscles is one of the most trusted ways of burning fat as it is believed that a pound of muscle can burn 6 calories of fat at rest while on the other hand a pound of fat burns 2 calories. Taking protein is another way to supplement because it has more thermogenic effect compared to the other macronutrients. Protein is always more hard to digest and as a result consume more energy in comparison to the carbs or fats. Another way to increase the BMR and having a healthy body is to keep taking meals at regular intervals as it increases the metabolism. Since the process of digestion consumes energy and each macro-nutrient has different proportions for the consumption of energy, so taking meals at regular intervals keeps the metabolism process active.

Taking fresh food is another way to keep the metabolic rate active. Foods which are closest to the natural form are always better compared to the processed foods that are pre-digested. Last but not the least; drinking water is the most effective ingredient to maintain a healthy and lean body. Not only does it flush out the fat from the body, it also helps the messaging systems to work correctly. It helps raising the metabolism and at the same time keeps the body balanced. Other factors which can help in raising the metabolic rates are drinking green tea, taking less stress and having proper sleep.

Reverse dieting is another way to help increase the metabolism as it increases the calorie intake slowly, day by day. The process is not about consuming calories suddenly; but it is a slow process wherein specific intake of calories is done week by week in an increasingly phased out manner. This process differs from person to person; but the guided theory remains the same.

Having a basic idea about how you can optimize your efforts for a fit and heathier body by boosting your metabolism and by following the right diet will help you gain the perfect physique in much less time!

DETOX: THE WAY INTO A BETTER HEALTH

I and Dustin have been in this fitness and health industry since 18 years and our mission is to remove the junk, which resides in the body. That is the reason our smoothie bar came into picture for conducting all the nutrition coaching and all the fitness related business from our gym space. This continued for 3 years until we started our in-person and online coaching. There cannot be any better inspiration than seeing your clients reach their goal and having their lives and health transformed. It's always good to see clients taking their ownership and growing in their practice of health and knowledge. All junks have been stripped off so that nothing but the best reached our customers, which is the non-toxic, the purest and the cleanest product possible.

The whey protein made from New Zealand does not contain majority of lactose for easing the process of digestion. We normally try to make the diet a perfect one to get that perfect body; but it should also be noted that no diet is the perfect diet at all times and in all cases. It really becomes very difficult to find if the products we are eating are actually consumable or not. For example; the sugar-free foods, which we take are chemically sweetened with a sweetener called as Splenda and the so-called fresh vegetables and fruits are genetically modified or sprayed with pesticides. The meat we buy is from the animals treated with antibiotics that help them to grow faster and even the tap water is full of arsenic, lead and mercury. A majority of all these chemicals that were created in the last couple of centuries with the latest technology and ever increasing knowledge has just changed everything that we used to call "fresh and pure" food.

Chemicals are there in each and every step of the processes, which lead the food to your table. The entire process starting from harvesting, producing and processing followed by packing the same in toxic plastics along with other packaging and finally to transporting – in each and every step the chemicals are added to the food.

Even the foods found on the shelves these days aren't food anymore. These are nothing but the storehouses of chemicals and some of them are described below:

- Acrylamide: It usually forms when food is fried or baked at high temperature and as the by-product of the cigarette smoke.

- Arsenic: It is found in many of the home-building products.
- Triclosan: It is used as the antibacterial agent in many of the personal care products such as hand soap and toothpaste.

While the body tissues have detoxification organs for processing most of these chemicals as well as toxins, any exposure to these chemicals can cause severe medical issues. It's nothing but a business where in more and more quantity of food is grown at a cheaper price and that too within a small span of time so that the accumulated profits can be very high. This is leading to adulteration. While I am particularly not against any one making any profits, but I am surely against the idea of making it a business at the cost of someone's health.

For an example, we all knew cows consume grass as their food; but these days many are feeding them with cheap grains just only to fatten them up. There are many issues with these and the most disgusting of all is that these grains are treated with pesticides, insecticides and herbicides or they are genetically modified. This diet is always very tough on the cattle's digestive system resulting in inflammatory issues. Every year, an estimated 15 million pounds of these antibiotics are used in the grains, which are fed to the cattle just to make them look fatter and bigger. These antibiotics get stored in their fats, which are finally consumed by the humans.

Let's come to the by-products of cattle that is milk. There are many growth hormones that are injected just to double the quantity of milk. While these hormones are banned in most of the countries, in many countries, it is still legal and to top it up, many farmers use it more than the prescribed limit.

Like these, there are many areas where the body picks up toxins and chemicals. The sources of these chemicals are mostly indirect to the body and are not realized practically. These days everyone has a different level of toxic overload or toxic burden. For instance, if someone has worked in a coal mine for years, he would surely have higher toxic levels than an average guy. He would have spent years inhaling toxic fumes than spending time taking vitamin D and that is why; his nutrition would also have gone for a toss. The moral is irrespective of the toxic level one carries, the goal is to minimize the intake of toxins into the body.

While the body is designed to filter out the chemicals on its own, the toxic levels of this era have been overwhelming and that's why, it needs a push from our side to keep ourselves fit and healthy. Health issues, diseases and complications can arise from the excess toxins present in the body. Our life, health and well-being depend on our dedication to flush out the toxicity from the body. While there are many toxic substances used in the food; none of these can kill us instantly. They act as a slow poison. They actually pose too much of undue burden on the kidneys, livers and other important organs. To learn more about the best detox programs, just *contact us and learn the best programs* to get rid of all toxins in your body.

To keep and maintain a healthy and wealthy life, it is important to first understand that we should know what we are eating. We should be aware of the differences between harmful choices and better choices. While it is very easy to just get overwhelmed with all this information, it is equally tough to practice it in real life. Minimizing the intake of toxic substances is all that is needed as the first step in this direction. While it is true that we can never be free of toxins, the best we can do is to minimize the quantity. And there may be many people who have plans of build their own houses without using any varnishes or wood stains; people who would plan to eating only from their own organic garden, gathering water only from a stream of fresh mountain, raising their own grass fed cattle, making their body wash and spinning their organic cotton for the personal clothing line are very small in number. We should do both: minimize the intake of toxins and maximize the elimination of these. That's why we should detox our body from head to toe as there is not a single body part which is not touched by the harmful toxins.

The first step in this direction is to take the right food as this will reach and affect the stomach and blood. Additionally, the kind of food supply we are receiving can adulterate the entire world with its big source of toxin. Though in the perfect world; non-processed, complete organic and home-grown foods are recommended; but the reality is that we are striving for progress and not perfection. In this scenario, even one decision of eliminating the toxins from the body is considered a win. For protein, grass fed beef is always recommended; but if it's fed on organic grass, it's always better. That clearly signifies that no hormones or antibiotics have been used for this. The cattle were pasture raised and were grazed on pesticide-free grass. This is very much important especially when we are in the fight for minimizing toxins from the body. The grass-fed beef is also rich in conjugated linoleic acid and omega 3. Cows are basically designed to consume grass; not grain. This is not only dangerous for the cow; but this acidic meat is then passed on to the end customer and so, the meat will not have the nutrient profile that it should ideally have. That is the reason; we should look for grass-fed organic beef. There are some phenomenal nutrients, which we get only from grass-fed beef. The same logic of beef applies to chicken. You may have seen an ad for an all-vegetarian diet fed to the cattle; but again that is not their natural diet. If it is not very much clear and explicit on the packaging, it is always better to ask for further clarity. In an ideal condition, a chicken diet is supposed to consist of insects and seeds; but if they are fed with vegetables, then we are questioning their natural diet. Vegetarian diets are nothing but marketing gimmick, which are used to sell their products.

Coming to eggs, they are undoubtedly one of the most confusing products because of the continuing and prevailing marketing shenanigans. An egg container can have close to 12 varieties of certifi-cations. While there are few which are useful, majority of them are useless. All the questions answers here for beefs can be easily related to the market trips of the farmer. We want chicken, which are fed organically; we want eggs, which are from these chickens; we want vegetables, which are grown without any pesticides and fertilizers and we want our body to be a system, which can actually flush out all toxic substances without realizing that all these involve a lot of study, research and hard work to understand the source and quality of food.

Even dairy products like cheese should be bought with caution. However, it is less likely that it will cause any diges-tive problem. When cheese is made, the bacteria turn the hard lactose into lactic acid and thus, the end product is always easier to digest. The product tends to be calorie dense and that's why we recom-mend it to be taken in smaller moderation. What we want is raw grass fed cheese and hence, the next best option would be organic cheese.

Another product, which misleads us, is soy protein. It has found its use in many products. While we are under the assumption that it's a good one; in real life, it's a very cheap product. Soy has many natural toxins and thus, is linked to many health conditions including impaired digestive system, impaired thyroid func-tion, prevention of absorption of certain minerals and a hormonal imbalance.

It is not only the animal prod-ucts and their indirect products, which contain toxins. Even fruits and vegetables are a part of the ecosystem. Vegetables which we eat are more likely to be grown using pesticides and other fertilizers and are present in the form of toxins in our body. It is our sole responsibility to check out the processes these vegetables and fruits have been grown under or at least know the source of these farms. Veggies are very low in calories and very high in nutrition and are thus very effective in providing an ideal balanced diet. They are actually a great way to fill the stomach especially when we are on a low calorie diet. To make the most of vegetables, it is recommended to have a chopper so that we can chop some of them and add to whatever food we want of our choice. We can even blend them in a blender with some other fruits and have shakes. Additionally, we may look up to new recipes and add them to our veggie regimen. And for some not-so-great news, on an average, we consume 4.5 billion pounds pesticides in a year. While the government may say that these are safe, the 8-9 varieties of them add on to make a humongous difference. This will have dangerous implication on the body.

There are many ways to keep the nutrient quantity in vegetables intact and one of them is to keep them in refrigerator. When organic veggies and fruits are frozen, it retains the nutrients. It is also recommended that these veggies are kept without cutting. There are many companies, which offer organic foods right at the door step.

Another item which is very rich in vitamins, minerals and other fats is nuts. Since balance of nutrient is essential, it is advisable to have proper content of omega 3 and omega 6 and in proper ratio. Most of the nuts have higher contents of omega 6 and so you should balance that out with those having omega 3 also. What you need to look out for is to have a ratio of 1:1. Thais will naturally help to avoid the toxins, chemicals and pesticides. You can have unsalted nuts to keep the sodium level intact. However, if they are salted with Himalayan salt or sea salt, that's perfectly fine. Coming to peanuts, they are not nuts; but actually belong to the legume family. So they are grown in ground and not on tree. However, it is always recommended to minimize their intake as they are grown in ground and they have a thin shell. Because of this, they are always exposed to toxic substances like insecticides and pesticides. They are also rich in omega 6 fatty acids. So, if peanut butter is a part of your diet, then this is surely a good sign.

Next comes the supplements, which are generally consumed to gain muscles. At the top of the chart is quality protein powder that contains a grass fed and whey protein powder. You also need to make sure that only sunflower lecithin is used and not the soy lecithin. Next comes multi vitamins, which are normally taken in the form of capsules and are composed of synthetic ingredients using binders and cheap fillers. Fish oil is also considered to be a very good health supplement for its multiple health benefits. Vitamin K and Vitamin D3 are next on the list. Though vitamin D3 is lacking in majority of the people and vitamin K helps in absorbing the same.

The last on the list is magnesium, which is consumed by over 300 processes; but still we lack the same in our body.

Well, this article has absorbed an in-depth analysis of various toxins and their effects on the body and the ways and means to minimize them. There is no shadow of doubt that if these points are kept in mind and followed well, the body will be less affected with toxins and will be healthier than ever. But it is always easier said than done. This demands a full dedication towards our health and a step by step procedure for monitoring the progress made. As far as possible, the focus should always be on organic products.

WHAT IS DETOX: INTRODUCTION

Today's is the age of contradictions. The human kind has achieved phenomenal progress, learnt to control many natural systems, eliminated killer diseases, raised the income and awareness levels of people across the world and in general, made the life much easier and safer than it was barely a hundred years back. But the flip side is that each individual has become more insecure, tensed, restless and unsure of everything.

Everyone is in a perpetual hurry, without really doing something beautiful, joyous or satisfying. Not just the mind, soul and the spirit; but also the body is filled with undesired elements. We experience fatigue and sickness without moving a limb, we develop skin problems, we suffer from headaches... More

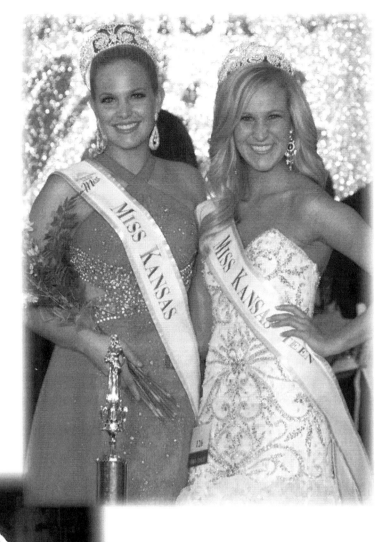

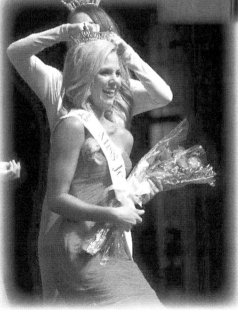

and more manual tasks in our daily life are now done by machines. We hardly ever walk now. We don't have to exert the body any more in our struggle for survival. We don't exercise the body at all. As a result, almost every person needs a regular detox operation to get the body and the mind back at their cheerful, refreshed and positive best.

People need to rest and recharge themselves every few weeks. They have to find time to relax, eat and drink healthy food to help the body to neutralize the ill-effects of the neglect over the past weeks and detox itself so that it can recover enough to resume the routine life. Detoxification involves resting, cleaning and nourishing the body. Detoxification is the physiological or medicinal removal of toxic substances from the human body. All that is toxic is removed from the body and it is refilled with healthy nutrients in processes devised and conducted by experts.

When the need for detoxification was felt and established, many detox procedures were developed quickly. In fact, the need for such detox was felt even much earlier. When the life was slow, it needed all people to exert physically to get through their daily routine. But detox, during those times, was neither so frequent nor so universal. People across the world developed their own ways to get over such lows and return refreshed to resume the struggle. Various relaxation and concentration techniques form a part of the detox process. Fasting, fruit juices and clean food have always had their place in human life. Alternative

medicine branches practice various types of detoxification, including detoxification diets. Many detox diets and detox courses suitable for specific cases are now run to get the people back to their very best, physically and mentally.

The number of detox followers is growing day by day and people are enjoying the multiple benefits provided by this unique process. We hope to provide information about the best ways to detox to maximize the health benefits.

THE BEST WAYS TO DETOX YOUR BODY

Detoxification methods and techniques have multiplied quickly over the past few years. These include exercises, cleansing diets, cleanse drinks and relaxation. Such courses aim at cleansing and rejuvenating the body completely. Detox also treats the mind and the soul. The basic idea is to remove all food from the body and increase the intake to water, fruits and vegetables for about a week. The routine food is then reintroduced slowly. A detox diet presents the liver with an opportunity to remove the backlog of toxins collected over a long period. This process purifies the body and enables it to return to its high efficiency levels.

ON LIQUID DIET

Most detox diets are low-calorie liquid foods. Fruit juices, vegetables and water dominate the detox diets. This means a greatly lightened load for the usually overburdened digestive system of the body. The body is regularly digesting saturated fats, proteins, salt and sugar, probably all of them in quantities more than necessary for the body. During the detox week, the body load is reduced and the entire backlog is cleared. The result is improved health and increased energy and vitality. Thus, a regular body detoxification proves to be an excellent preventative measure that promotes the general health.

Various detox programs achieve body purification by providing an opportunity for the digestive organs to rest through the fasting period, by encouraging the liver to push the toxins out of the system and to spur toxin removal through intestines, kidneys and skin.

DO IT ONCE A YEAR

Various detox agencies recommend that everyone should undergo the detoxification process once every year. It is good for persons with symptoms of unexplained fatigue, skin Irritation, recurring allergies, mental confusion and menstrual problems. Persons intending to go for a detox procedure should stop taking liquor, smoking, sugars and coffee a few days earlier. They should also reduce their exposure to household cleansers, shampoos, deodorants and toothpastes. They should use the natural substitutes for all these products. They also should avoid the potential situations of tension and stress.

THE BEST DETOX PROGRAM

Most detoxification agencies have different detox programs for people with different needs. Many agencies design a detox program to suit the needs of each person. They have many ready recipes suitable for individuals with specific problems. The best among the detox programs follow a week-long schedule. On the first two days, the intake allowed is merely liquids. The next five-day diet helps the digestive system to rest. This diet includes fresh fruit and vegetable juices and water.

DO THIS AND LIVE WELL

Post-detoxification, you can keep cleansing the body daily with the inclusion of a lot of fiber and fresh fruits and vegetables of all types like beet, radish, cabbage and broccoli in the diet. Drink green tea and two liters of water a day. Besides this, concentration on positive emotions, regular deep breathing exercise and yoga exercises for an hour will help you achieve your target. It will also be useful for the body to have a five-minute hot shower followed by cold water for 30 seconds. The process should be repeated thrice. This should end in rest in bed for half an hour.

FOODS THAT CAN HELP IN EFFECTIVE DETOXIFICATION

The body-mind link is real at least in case of good food. If the body is well-fed and content, the mind works smoothly, positively and creatively. The food we consume must be free of toxins and free radicals. Regular exercise, healthy diet and rejection of alcohol and sugars do wonders. Some foods have natural cleansing properties. If they are a part of our regular diet all the time, they can help to remove the toxic remains of the other food you may be partaking from time to time. Here is a list of the healthy, clean food.

- **Onion:** Healthy and tasty, onion has amino acids, which promotes the liver cleansing process. Beneficial red onions lose 20 percent of quercetin and 75 percent of anthocyanins. Onions absorb arsenic, cadmium, lead, mercury and tin in foods. They trigger the body's inflammatory responses.

- **Garlic:** It strengthens the immune system and bolsters liver functions. It adds to the flavor of the food.

- **Ginger:** It offers many health benefits. It is also added in tea and many foods. It boosts the functioning of the liver and has some astringent properties.

- **Lemons:** Lemons and lemon juice are instrumental in flushing the toxins out of the body. Lemon juice is added to water and consumed. It may be flavored with pepper. A cup of hot water with lemon juice prepares the digestive system for the day's work.

- **Apples;** Apples provide fiber, vitamins, minerals, D-glucarate, flavonoids and terpenoids.

Flavonoids stimulate the bile output and rid the liver of some toxins. Apples have a soluble fiber called pectin, which removes metals and food additives from the body.

- **Almonds:** It is the best nut source of vitamin E, with each ounce containing 7.3 mg of alpha-tocopherol vitamin E. They also provide fiber, calcium, magnesium and protein that stabilize the blood sugar levels.

- **Coriander:** It contains many antioxidants and pushes mercury and metals out of the tissue. Its antibacterial action kills salmonella.

- **Pineapple:** Its digestive enzyme, bromelain, cleanses the colon and improves the digestion. It reduces excessive inflammation, prevents the coagulation of blood and stops the growth of certain tumors.

- **Cabbage:** Its diuretic properties help to get rid of excess liquids in the body and take away toxins with it. Sulfur-rich cabbage assists the liver in breaking down toxins and expelling them easily. Sulfur detoxifies free radicals and reactivates the oxygen species.

- **Turmeric:** Drinking turmerictea for a week can by itself detox the body.

- **Water:** Water is vital for all of organs and also for flushing the toxins. After exercise and saunas, take more water to remain hydrated.
- **Asparagus:** It helps in fighting the aging processes, protects you from cancer and helps the heart to remain healthy.
- **Beet**: Beet helps to destroy the free-radicals, thus joining the forces against cancer.
- **Broccoli**: It works with enzymes in liver to turn toxins into compounds that the body can remove easily.
- **Green tea**: It has high antioxidant value. It kills free radicals and prevents harm to the body.
- **Lemongrass**: It helps the liver, kidneys, bladder and the digestive tract. Its consumption leads to improved circulation, good digestion and a better complexion.
- **Watercress**: It releases liver enzymes that help the liver to get rid of toxins. Regular watercress consumption fights breast cancer.
- **Wheatgrass**: It means a big boost for the liver. It lowers blood sugar and gets the metabolism back on normal.
- **Grapefruit**: It has fiber and nutrient-rich juice. It fills the body with good things and removes the bad things. It helps in quick weight loss.
- **Cinnamon**: Its oil has cinnamaldehyde, cinnamyl acetate and cinnamyl alcohol. Cinnamaldehyde prevents clumping of the blood cells. It is an anti-microbial food. It stops the growth of bacteria and fungi. It has high antioxidant value.
- **Fennel**: It is high in fiber and useful in preventing colon cancer. Fennel provides folate necessary to breakdown homocysteine into benign molecules. Its vitamin C is antimicrobial and is required for the proper functioning of the immune system.
- **Flaxseeds**: Ground flaxseeds provide the fiber that binds and flushes toxins from the intestine. They also provide omega 3 oils. Flax fiber reduces appetite and boosts weight loss.
- **Hemp**: Hemp is full of vitamins E and C and chlorophyll that cleanse the body. The soluble and insoluble fiber in hemp keeps the digestive tract clean.
- **Basil**: It has anti-bacterial properties and is rich in antioxidants. It backs the kidneys and helps the body to expel toxins. It has anti-ulcer properties and anti-microbial effects that help in fighting bacteria, yeast, fungi and mold.

While all these are good foods for detox, there are some foods that have to be avoided. They include alcohol, caffeinated drinks, sweets, chocolates and overeating.

WHAT YOU SHOULD NOT DO DURING DETOXIFICATION PROCESS

The detox program is supposed to rejuvenate the body, not create more problems for it. So people, who collect a lot of toxins in their bodies because of the faulty lifestyles and individual prefer-ences, cannot switch over to the ideal diet in a jiffy. They have to prepare the body for the changes and act in such a way that the body gets used to them. This will take time and the persons concerned will have to be patient. There are many things people should not do in connection with the entire detox mission.

- Avoid foods that obstruct the detox process. Do not consume dishes with added sugars, which hinder the production of the necessary enzymes.
- Avoid alcohol. Even small amounts can ruin the detox procedure.
- Avoid more than a cup of coffee a day. If you cannot do this immediately, do this gradually.
- Digestion of dairy products means a heavy burden on the detoxification system. So keep milk, cheese and yoghurt away.

- Avoid eating things having monosodium glutamate (MSG) or modified food starch, carrageenan, glutamic acid and hydrolyzed vegetable protein.
- Do not consume packaged foods like soups, vegetables, cereals, and cookies. They contain salts, preservatives, flavors, sweeteners and fats; but no healthy nutrients.
- Do not use fruits and vegetables for cooking or eating without washing them thoroughly.
- Do not eat them without peeling.
- Do not eat too much of meat if your body cannot handle it easily.
- Avoid white rice, pasta, potatoes and white breads.
- Keep away from trans-fats. Fried and packaged snacks, doughnuts, cookies, fast food and cakes contain trans-fat.
- Avoid products with gluten to reduce the workload on the liver.
- Pregnant or lactating women should not go for a detox program because their needs of calcium, protein and iron are almost doubled. They will have a shortage of this if they go in for a detox program.
- Pregnant women should not opt for a detox program also because the toxins released in the process are mixed with the

blood. These may be carried to the fetus and affect its health.

- If you decide to change your eating habits, do not change the diet abruptly. Go about it in a slow, gradual way, allowing the body to get adjusted to the change.

WHAT YOU MUST DO

A detox program will produce better results when your mind and body are at peace. So, spare a few minutes every day for relaxation, meditation and for finalizing your goals. A professional massage a day before the detox program should do the body a lot of good. Make it a point to remain active before and during detox.

DETOX FOREVER

A regular annual detox program, however meticulous, should not act as a license for an eating and drinking orgy for the rest of the year. The detoxification of the body has to continue around the year at a practically possible level to ensure that the body remains in the best possible state.

SOME MYTHS ABOUT DETOXIFICATION THAT MUST BE BUSTED

The detox industry is growing pretty fast. More and more people, including celebrities, are opting for it. The advertisement blitz continues 24X7 and more people are tempted to try the magical results promised. The scientific opinion about detox is pure and simple skepticism. If the over-indulgence by people in fast food, smoking and alcohol is cured by one-time, one-week detox program, it is godsend for all such people, who form a huge majority across the world.

IT'S A FRAUD

The science proponents are never tired of saying that the idea that someone can flush the impurities from the body and rejuvenate the organs after a week-long session is a fraud. They say it is a clever ploy to sell things to the gullible people. The detox concept is a myth, they affirm. Business companies and quacks have conspired together to sell a bogus treatment that claims to remove the accumulated toxins from the body, say the science representatives.

NO DETOX CAN IMPROVE BODY FUNCTIONING

They point out that the body will need some serious medical attention if it accumulates toxins. Kidneys, liver, skin and lungs keep removing toxins all the time. No detox program can make them work better. The science community says the detox industry claims that toxins make their way into the body through food, air and water pollution but nobody spells out what exactly the toxins are. Nobody measures the level of each toxin before the detox program and after. No manufacturer of detox product can present some evidence of the efficacy of any of their long list of costly products. The pro-science group is positive that everything about the detox industry is a myth. Nothing of it is true, they assert.

There are more myths connected with the detox industry.

- According one, detoxing is the fastest way to lose weight. Detoxing does lose weight quickly, but you regain more than the lost kilograms in quick time once the procedure ends and you go back to your normal diet. And there is a limit to losing the weight. You can lose more weight slowly by following the traditional methods.

- It is also claimed that detox diets are better than the regular diet and exercise routine. Detox diets do remove some toxins, but it is easier and safer to opt for regular diet and exercise.

- There is a common impression that detox diets do not require any exercise. You do lose weight when on a detox diet without exercise, but you also lose muscle. If you wish to retain muscle, you have to exercise.

- It is believed that detox diets have strange juices and minimal food intake. Healthy detox foods do not need expensive juices. Detox foods can be made by anyone using lemons, green leafy vegetables, sesame seeds and green tea.

- They say that excessive water consumption detoxes the body. Water does spur the function of the liver and kidneys, but extra water leads to side effects like headaches, nausea and disorientation.

- Another myth is that you can use sauna as a detox. Saunas do release toxins from the skin after a workout, but that is not because of the detox program. Long periods in sauna may also lead to dehydration. It may also affect the body's ability to detoxify over time.

Although the scientific opinion is explicitly holding all the detox programs as a huge hoax, the popularity of these programs is zooming up. The detox industry claims that the toxic levels in today's lifestyle and era of pollution are so high that the body cannot remove all the toxins on its own. It needs help to achieve that. The detox programs are the right answer for the prevailing situation, they claim.

CONCLUSION

A cursory glance at most of the detoxification programs reveals that there is hardly anything new in them. People all over the word have been fasting regularly with a view to putting a lesser burden on the body organs periodically. Consumption of fruit juices or vegetable soups had also been common among almost all the communities across the world. People kept away from alcohol too on such days. The modern detoxification programs are variations of these. Some of the variations are thoughtful, some gimmicks and some clearly aimed at misleading the client into accepting them and pay for them.

IS IT A FRAUD OR A GIMMICK?

Whether the contention of science that the detoxification programs are nonsense, fraud and gimmicks is true or not, more and more people are opting for it. They are ready to pay substantially high amounts for the programs. And the most important thing about the programs is that the people do not seem to be regretting the decision. They are getting a lot of benefits out of the programs and they obviously think that they are getting their money's worth. If that is so, no one can stop them.

BODY IS UNDER MORE STRAIN

It is absolutely clear that the modern lifestyle is putting a lot more strain on the body than in the recent past. Most of what we eat is not healthy. Much of what we consume is positively unhealthy. With the incomes of the lower strata of countries across the world going up steeply, more people are eating fried snacks, fast food, sweets, dairy products, alcohol, tobacco and meats of various types. Although the body is capable of handling all such stuff, there is a good chance that it may be overloaded most of the time and could be in need of some respite. It may welcome some rest in the form of a detox program. Hence, nothing can please the stressed people of the world more than being able to participate in a detoxification program recommended by the experts.

THE IMPORTANCE OF MENTAL HEALTH AND THE MIND OF A CHAMPION

No feeling can match the feeling of winning. To taste this feeling, you need to come out of your comfort zone and do some back breaking hard work to get complete control over your body and mind. The author, Patricia Payne, is recognized all around the world as the best female bodybuilder (that too drug-free) in the world. As a kid, she was a sports lover. TV never attracted her as much as sports did. She started towards her goal of a fit body in her twenties and displayed good results. When she turned 30, she switched to Gold's Gym. She barely ate and ran some 5 miles a day. Ultimately she got a zero figure; but felt miserable. So, she hired a trainer and gained some real muscles.

Hosting a perfect body, one of her friends asked her if she was in for a competition. She refused. But being pushed on by her friend, she walked up the ramp, in a tiny bikini and won the competition. And since then, she has never turned back. This whole process has not just been about body building and developing muscles but building confidence and strength - the strength to drive the best out of you.

She describes the entire process as relying on the three pillars: utter commitment, strong willpower and remaining motivated.

She then describes the reason for taking a natural route to bodybuilding rather than resorting to any drugs. Using the latter leads to bad health and doesn't go with the spirit of sportsmanship and athletics. That is why; she preferred to put in double the amount of hard work, paying proper attention to her nutrition and adopted the natural way to bodybuilding.

WHAT YOU BELIEVE IS WHAT YOU ARE

The author says that what you tell yourself every time you cross a mirror or every time you win/lose or every time you wake up is true and that is what you believe from within. This is the part of the inner dialogue. Your conscience will never lie to you. The inner you knows exactly what you can achieve and what you can't. And you choose what you believe! If you don't think good about yourself, you will always end up in having a lower self-esteem and this might lead you to make wrong choices. Self-limiting beliefs are even dangerous as they prevent you from achieving the zenith and thus living your life to the full potential. So before venturing into something new, you need to stop and ask yourself the belief as to why you want to or you don't want to do a certain thing.

The source of beliefs is somewhere buried deep in your childhood days. But such beliefs may be right or wrong. And to get over the wrong beliefs is not an easy task. You need to identify the wrong ones and challenge them fiercely. As changing beliefs can open up new paths for you and you may become more positive and start thinking and acting differently.

Just remember it all starts with the mind. If you wish to bring out the hidden champion within you, you know where to start now.

CONFIDENCE IS THE KEY!

As said earlier, the mind is the place where the manifestation of a strong will to do something great takes place; one can't have a strong mind if he lacks confidence. To build confidence, you should let go of all your fears and ego.

WITH SELF-CONFIDENCE COMES SELF-RESPECT WHICH IF FOLLOWED BY SUCCESS.

For building confidence you should be aware of your strengths as well as weaknesses. You should take out some-time to talk to yourself, observe your actions, know your emotions and then act accordingly. Next, you should learn how to manage your fears. All fears are not bad. After all, they protect you from anything bad happening to you. But fears like fear of failure, fear of embarrassment and fear of rejection should be shun outright.

Surprisingly, there is also a fear of success. One might fear of being lonely when he achieves what he wanted. But again, this is as harmful as the previous three and should be overcome.

THE ROLE OF WILLPOWER!

Willpower is defined as a response in the sense that the reaction comes from an inner conflict. This means that if you want to do something, say bunk your gym for a day, but you know you shouldn't do it, this becomes an inner conflict. This is where your willpower comes into action. In dilemmas like these, your willpower will provide you a just solution. You can use your willpower more wisely once you learn to manage your stress levels, focus better and get good amount of sound sleep. You can manage stress by taking short breaks and engaging into some fun filled activities.

Stress usually leads to fatigue and the best way to overcome fatigue is to sleep. A good 7 to 8 hour sleep can do wonders in your life. As when you will wake up, you will be energetic and be able to think afresh, right from the scratch.

And don't forget that a focused mind is a healthy mind. You can do yoga and other exercises, which can keep you more focused.

JUST RELISH YOUR DIET!

Always remember if you are not enjoying what you are doing, then it is not worth it.

As far as your diet is concerned, it is your attitude towards your diet, which matters. This attitude is comprised of the motives and the beliefs for you choosing this diet. The three possible attitudes are:

1. **All or Nothing thinking.**
    This consists of diet, which is too harsh to follow. If you are carrying this attitude, then you will end up being disappointed. All or nothing diets are the ones, which will make you starve. But how long will you be able to continue this? A week? A month? It's an impossible task at hand.

2. **The ultimate sacrifice:**
    If you think you are sacrificing your food for the sake of shedding some extra pounds, you are mistaken, my friend. If you starting off at such a negative note, how can you think to last long in the battle?

3. **The ultimate chaos:**
    This is exactly opposite to the previous one. The ultimate chaos happens when you keep on switching or adding or subtracting elements from your diet. Say you follow two meals a day for two days and then switch to three meals a day! It is nothing but an utter chaos which will lead you nowhere.

All in all, the above three should be given up immediately. Just move on and learn from your mistakes. The one and the only way to achieve your goal is to commit to that goal. Once you have committed, nothing can take you away from it. We offer courses, *distant as well as online*, to those who would love to learn about this in death and derive maximum benefits from this.

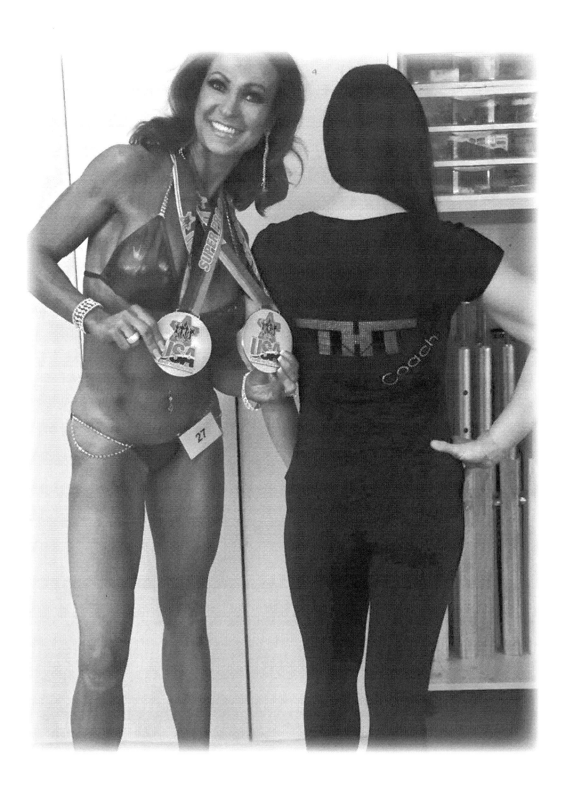

INTRODUCTION: WHY IS IT IMPORTANT TO CONTROL BLOOD PRESSURE AND CHOLESTEROL?

Well, the terms 'Blood Pressure' and 'Cholesterol' must be sounding very common to you these days. But I doubt if anyone knows the actual meaning of it. Many people have a misconception that they are clear with these two terms; but in reality, they hardly know what the actual meaning is.

WHAT IS BLOOD PRESSURE AND CHOLESTEROL?

Blood Pressure is the pressure exerted in the process of blood circulation upon the walls of the blood vessels. It is measured at the person's upper arm.

Cholesterol is a type of fat that is found in our blood and is necessary to help our skin, brain and all the other organs to grow and work properly.

Nowadays, the majority of the population is seen suffering from high blood pressure and increased cholesterol levels, which is not a sign of a healthy body. They do not understand the importance of having accurate blood pressure and cholesterol level in the human body. Taking such major issues for granted

is the root cause for several diseases. If proper care is taken, then such problems would never arise and the person can remain free from diseases.

A healthy person should have 120/80 mm Hg of blood pressure. This statistical figure in your report is the proof that you are taking good care of yourself and are on the right track to avoid any disease. On the other hand, an ideal ratio for the cholesterol level is less than 3.5 to 1. A higher ratio than this is not considered to be good for the human body and thus, may be the cause for your frequent visits to the doctor.

Because of the busy schedule, many people cannot pay much attention to their health and this is the reason that they are unaware about the importance of such things in their life. One should know why it is necessary for a human body to have controlled blood pressure and cholesterol levels. Here are the reasons:

- **Being more energized**
  If you have a high Cholesterol level in your body, you will definitely feel lethargic and inattentive for the entire day. The day would become over-tiring and slowly and gradually,

you will not be able to do your work properly. On the other hand, if the blood pressure and cholesterol levels are accurate, the body remains fit and energized. The activeness can be clearly seen and the person can enjoy the working because his physical condition allows doing so.

- **Reduced risk of heart diseases**
  This is one of the most important reasons, for a person to have an accurate degree of cholesterol and blood pressure in his or her body. Inappropriate ratios will definitely be a major factor for you becoming ill very often. The heart diseases get a push when you have high cholesterol in your body. Do consider it a serious issue and act accordingly.

- **Mood Swings**
  If at all, you are physically unfit, because of your inexact ratios, then it is bound to be reflected in your behavior and way of talking. If you are not active and comfortable to sit and chat with your friends, you start acting rude and these mood swings are of great harm to your social, personal and professional life. This is one of the reasons, why people should have a low blood pressure and cholesterol level.

Do not take your health condition so lightly, because it is a matter of utmost importance. Understand the need of the hour and take appropriate measures to maintain a proper health. If you know that you are the victim of a high blood pressure or high cholesterol level, then do not wait further. Visit a doctor and start taking the precautions from today itself. Understand the importance of controlled blood pressure and cholesterol in the human body and take immediate actions.

DIFFERENT WAYS TO CONTROL BLOOD PRESSURE AND CHOLESTEROL

Very often, it is seen that even after knowing that you have become the victim of high or low blood pressure or cholesterol level, you do not pay much attention to the issue. This can happen because of two reasons; either the person does not have enough time to go and visit the doctor and take the required precautions or he or she lacks knowledge about what to do and what not to do to keep the blood pressure and cholesterol in control. If the case happens to be the former one, then the person is utterly careless about his or her health. On the other hand, if the person does not have proper information about the precautions to take, then he need not worry much, for the advanced medical science nowadays, is a great support for such people.

In order to achieve the target of having controlled blood pressure and cholesterol, there are many things, which need to be kept in mind. To lead a healthy life, you need to follow some strict rules which will help you to achieve your desired target and prevent any heart disease or stroke in future.

- **Get Trim**
  Simply, it means to lose weight, if at all you are the victim of obesity. If you lose at least 5 to 10 percent of your body weight, it will surely help you in maintaining a proper cholesterol level and suitable blood pressure. Your body will work with more energy and mental awareness. You will feel like doing work with more concentration and interest and thus, the quality of your work will also increase.

- **Exercise daily**
  Well, this can be called the mantra to remain fit. As per the medical research, if you exercise daily for at least 30 minutes, you can surely bring down your blood pressure to a normal level and also improve the cholesterol levels. Just keep yourself moving and there will be no chance of becoming the victim of any health problem.

- **Eat bananas**
  As is said, eating too much of salt raises the blood pressure to a very high level, which obviously is not good for the body. Eating a banana a day will raise your potassium extent, which neutralizes the ill effects of sodium. Hence, it is highly beneficial.

- **Cut Salt**
  Those who have extremely high blood pressure should avoid eating salt as much as possible, for it is really harmful for them. Whenever you eat labelled foods, do not forget to check their sodium content. It is a precaution that is advised by every doctor to a patient, for it has been proven medically that high sodium content in the body, harms the body. Eat less of salt to remain fit and fine.

- **Do not Smoke**
  The presence of tobacco and nicotine in the cigarettes is one of the reasons for a high blood pressure. Quit smoking, if you do not want to get stuck into such health related issues. Also, there are number of other health benefits that you can gain once you give up on your bad habit of smoking. Think over it!

Though the above-mentioned points may be difficult to practice in the real life, you must keep in mind that if you really want to get away with such problems and control your blood pressure and cholesterol levels, you have no other option left. As the saying goes, 'a stich in time saves nine'. Therefore, do not wait for the right day to come and just start off today itself. No delays should be made, when the matter is about your health. Start changing your habits from today and be assured that gradually you will get used to it. You can reach us at to *buy the most effective supplements* that will help you achieve your goals.

FOODS THAT HELP TO CONTROL BLOOD PRESSURE AND CHOLESTEROL LEVEL

What you eat always has an impact on your health. There are certain foods which suits only a particular body. If your blood pressure is relatively high and you do not want to make the condition worse, there are certain foods which should be consumed. Same is the case for the cholesterol levels. Changing what you eat can really help you a lot if done with proper care and seriousness. It will be difficult at the first start; but slowly and gradually, you will develop a habit of the same and the things would automatically turn out to be easy.

Alter what you eat according to your physical health and just see the wonders! Well, many people are not aware of what type of food should be consumed in order to achieve the target of controlled blood pressure and cholesterol levels. This turns out to be a huge hurdle for them, in the process of remaining fit and vigorous. To put an end to all the confusion, here we have the list of some food items which should be consumed in or-der to attain the accurate blood pressure and cholesterol level:

- **Oats**
  Including oats in your daily meal, while benefit you with improved level of cholesterol and blood pressure. The oats are easily available in the market and can be consumed at any time of the day, preferably morning. They are considered to be light for the body and also do not have excess of fat content or calories.

- **Watermelon**
  An amino acid called, L-Citrulline, is present in this fruit, which is medically proven to be good to reduce high blood pressure. You must have noticed that the doctors suggest the high blood pressure patients to eat watermelon at least once in two days. It is rich in Vitamin A and potassium. Add this juicy fruit to your diet and see the results yourself. I bet you, you will be amazed on seeing the effects!

- **Sunflower seeds**
  Being rich in fiber, proteins and folic acid, the Sunflower seeds are considered to be one of the best foods for maintaining a proper ratio of blood pressure and cholesterol in the body. There is just one caution attached with the same: buy it without salt, to

reduce your sodium intake, otherwise it would turn out to be harmful, rather than helpful.

- **Oranges**

  Opt for a fresh orange or the fresh juice, once a day and see the magic. It is highly rich in nutrients and fiber and is best for the high blood pressure patients. It adds taste as well as nutrition to your diet.

  So, do not forget to buy the oranges whenever you visit the market. The pulpy fruit must be included in your diet from today itself!

- **Carrots**

  Regulate your heart and kidney functions by eating a carrot every day. Carrot juice is the best cure for everything. Just a simple exercise: take a carrot and east it up and you are done! That is it. Do not be lazy for this simple activity and include it in your daily routine to maintain a proper blood pressure and cholesterol level.

Prevention is better than cure. Follow this saying and do prevent yourself from visiting the doctor. Take a proper diet from today and avoid eating medicines in future. Do not waste your time in just thinking; rather get up and start all at once. It is rightly said; Health is Wealth. Therefore, do not let go this precious wealth from your hands and take proper care of it. You never know what happens next. Hence, take extra care from now.

THINGS TO AVOID FOR MAINTAINING YOUR BLOOD PRESSURE AND CHOLESTEROL LEVELS

Do you have a high blood pressure or low cholesterol level? Well, you are not alone. There are billions of people who suffer from high blood pressure and high cholesterol levels, yet they do not take proper care of themselves. The main reason for the same is that they are not aware about the causes of the same. Once they know the root cause for their high cholesterol or blood pressure; an immediate action can be taken.

The advanced medical research nowadays has simplified the matters to a large extent. Visiting the doctor and taking the precautions given by him, is not a difficult task. But why to let this happen? Stop any such problem at the first hand and avoid any visit to the doctor. There are certain DONT'S that should be strictly followed by a person in order to control the levels of blood pressure and cholesterol so as to lead a healthy and happy life.

- **Fast Foods**

  A very common habit that almost every person on this planet has is the habit of eating a lot of fast food. The junk food is the main cause of your poor health conditions because of the fats and excessive oil it contains, which is not at all good for the body. Do not eat the outside food very often and avoid it as much as possible. Include only the nutritious food in your diet and then see the results.

- **Reduce the activity level**
  The less your exercise, the more you are prone to these health related issues. Just get off the couch and give your body a move. It will not harm you at any cost. Do not ever reduce your outdoor activities at any cost, for they may really turn out to be very dangerous. Plan your day accordingly and set your priorities wisely.

- **Alcohol**
  Say a big NO to alcohol. Even if you drink occasionally, it will harm you at a later stage in life. Quit this habit of yours if you want to lead a healthy and tension-free life. Otherwise, be prepared to face the consequences.

- **Limit your Coffee**
  Well, if you have either high blood pressure or cholesterol level, then this is the time to kick off your frequent coffee habit. Just say a nice goodbye to the morning and evening coffee cups and change this daily routine of drinking coffee as soon as possible. Coffee includes soda and caffeine which are not good for the human body, if consumed in large extent. So take the right decision quickly!

- **Stress**
  If you are a patient of high blood pressure or high cholesterol level, then you should not get yourself into much stress. Try to stay away from the situations that make you feel stressed out and depressed. Keep your mood light and happy the entire day.

The above mentioned points should not be taken lightly, for they are of utmost importance. If you are serious about your health, then nobody can stop you from achieving your target. Focus on what you want and do not worry about the rest. Though, the habits are difficult to change all of a sudden; if efforts are made with full dedication and determination, there will be no difficulty. Health should be considered a top priority these days, because if you are not healthy, you will not be able to stand in this fast moving world.

Blood Pressure and cholesterol levels are not minor issues any longer, for these turn into huge diseases at a later stage. As is rightly said,' Prevention is better than cure'. Take the suitable measures beforehand and avoid any harm to your health.

CONCLUSION

A healthy outside, starts from the inside. Well, this is rightly said. If you want to outshine others and work wonders in your life, your physical fitness will play a very important role in doing so. No matter how good looking you are or how much wealth you acquire; if you are not in the condition to outcast your talent in front of the other people, then anything that you possess is of no use.

In this rat-race of earning money and fame, people forget that they are not machines, but a human being who needs proper care and rest. Irregular meals, fast foods, alcohol consumption, lack of physical exercise and many such factors are the root cause for the illnesses of the people. According to a latest survey conducted, the percentage of people having high blood pressure has risen from 38% to 79%. Such a huge rise is a clear sign of the carelessness that we human beings show towards our health and wellbeing.

We should set our priorities in such a manner that our fitness should not suffer at any cost. If need arises, a time table should be made which must include at least half an hour of physical workout, which can actually help us to attain normal levels of cholesterol and blood pressure.

Lose weight if you think you are becoming the victim of obesity, because even this turns out to be one of the reasons for people having high blood pressure. Exercise daily and that too with full interest and dedication. Anything which is not done with pleasure is almost a waste of time.

Include green vegetables in your diet and say NO to oily food to improve your cholesterol levels. Stop eating fried stuff and also the street food. Prefer green vegetables, salad, cereals and such light foods which are rich is fiber and protein.

Fruits should be included in the daily meal to improve your blood pressure level.

Heart diseases and stroke find their way through high blood pressure and cholesterol levels. If you do not take care of yourself at the first stage, then you are likely to become the victim of any such disease.

Go for regular health checkups and give yourself some time from your busy schedule. Continuous stress and overload of work also contribute to your bad health conditions.

Make a commitment from today onwards to include everything that is recommended by the doctor in your daily routine. Be it food or workout or whatever…Treat your doctor as your guru and follow him like a disciple. Only if you show determination and dedication, you can achieve your target. Otherwise, the process turns out to be very monotonous, especially when not done with interest and enjoyment.

If you are addicted to alcohol and any kind of drugs, stop them at once! Nothing is more important than your health. Visit a health expert and he will let you know the way to get rid of your addiction.

It is you who will be the reason for your health condition. It lies in your hands whether you want to lead a happy and healthy life in future, or want to just lie on the bed and wait for your death; Nobody else will help you to decide what you should do and what not. Good health is not something that you can buy, it needs to be earned. And the best way to earn it is to follow what the doctor says or the experts recommend.

Normal Blood pressure and cholesterol levels are very much important for your body to be fit. If at all, any ups or downs are noticed with these, a serious action should be taken. Do not let these issues be pending, for it may cost you a lot later. Take the right step today itself. Hurry up!

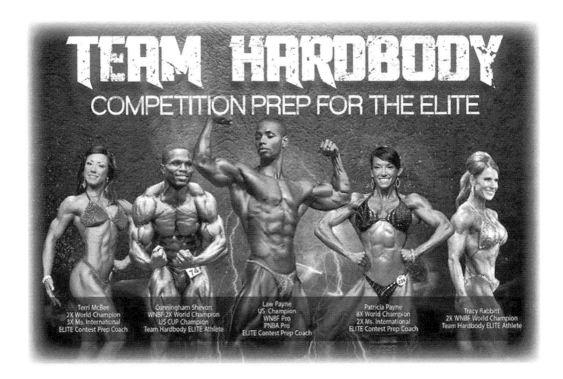

CONNECT WITH US, STAY IN TOUCH!

FOLLOW US ON:

Twitter:
https://twitter.com/lawpayne

Facebook:
https://www.facebook.com/LawPayneFitnessLLC/
https://www.facebook.com/thehardbodyteam/
https://www.facebook.com/PatriciaBeckman6xWorldChampionDrugFree4Life/

Instagram:
https://www.instagram.com/lawpaynefitnessonline/
https://www.instagram.com/8xworldchampion/
https://www.instagram.com/thehardbodyteam/

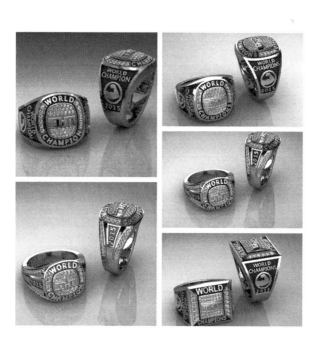

Made in the USA
Middletown, DE
04 June 2017